Praise for *Optimistic Aging*

Winner of the 2015 Independent Publisher's Living Now Book Award

"Dr. Henderson has indeed written an optimistic and practical roadmap to better health and aging. Her years of guiding others through lifestyle change are evident in her easy-to-use planning guide. A one-sitting and then a keep-handy book with valuable pearls."
— **Roger Landry, MD, MPH,** President of Masterpiece Living and author of *Live Long, Die Short: A Guide to Authentic Health and Successful Aging*

"Retirement planning should include a focus upon health in addition to financial security. Optimistic Aging provides an accessible guide to the non-financial aspects of retirement preparation."
— **Ronald Pressman,** Executive Vice President and Chief Operating Officer of TIAA-CREF

"Dr. Henderson is truly an academic who breaks down 'ivory tower' ideas to a practical constructive format that all of us can learn and grow from. Furthermore, *Optimistic Aging's* true gift comes from how otherwise unsavory aspects of aging are turned into zesty learning experiences, which are colorful and engaging. Dr. Henderson woos the reader into optimism!"
– **Chad Prusmack, MD,** Department of Neurosurgery, Rocky Mountain Spine Clinic

"*Optimistic Aging* is a practical guide to aging well. While it is crucial to save money for retirement to support our lifestyle, it is equally important to invest in our health to enjoy life fully. Margit reminds us that it's never too late to make healthy choices to improve our wellness. This is a must read to review and update annually."
– **Kimberly Curtis,** President and CEO of Wealth Legacy Institute, Inc., author of *Money Secrets: Keys to Smart Investing*

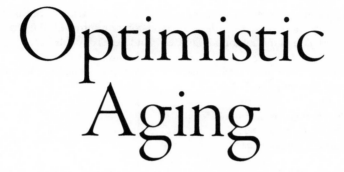

Optimistic Aging

from Midlife to the Good Life

~an Action Plan~

Margit Cox Henderson, Ph.D.

Resilient Publications

Optimistic Aging: from Midlife to the Good Life – an Action Plan
by Margit Cox Henderson, Ph.D.

Books may be purchased in quantity and/or special sales by contacting the author or publisher at
Resilient Publications
1805 S. Bellaire St., Suite 175
Denver, Colorado 80222
margit@margithenderson.com

Cover and Interior Design: Nick Zelinger (NZ Graphics)
Editing: All in the Proof and BTDT Enterprises

Library of Congress Control Number: 2014910917
ISBN: 978-0-9905189-0-7 (soft cover)
ISBN: 978-0-9905189-1-4 (e-book)

First Edition

Printed in the USA

Disclaimer:
The information presented in this book is intended to provide research-based guidance about aging well. Research offers conclusions drawn from group averages that may not be applicable in every individual case. Thus, the findings discussed herein are not a substitute for advice from a medical professional. The author and publisher specifically disclaim any and all liability arising directly or indirectly from the use or application of any information contained in this book. Be sure to consult a health care professional for medical advice about your specific situation.

For Gretl Cox and Bill Cox,
my aging-well inspirations

Contents

Preface

It is probably not a coincidence that the first words written in this book were while wearing my first pair of trifocal eyeglasses. I began this research project in my mid-40s. Feeling the impact of aging upon my own body and mind, I wanted to know how best to take care of myself going forward. Watching older loved ones age and die, witnessing their vulnerability and resilience, left me wondering what is in store for me.

This led me to read, read, and read some more. When discussing these findings with friends, all of them said they wanted to hear more about what I was learning. This prompted me to consider sharing these discoveries more formally.

I am not a gerontologist or a specialist on aging. My doctorate is in clinical psychology, and my strengths include literature review and synthesis as well as extensive knowledge about emotional and social health from over 20 years as a psychologist. I have no affiliation with the studies cited here, just a ravenous curiosity about what is known about aging well. As a researcher and teacher of research methods, I enjoy reading the detailed accounts of studies on aging. But most people don't have the time or interest to read at that depth. So I decided to write a succinct and user-friendly summary of the most robust findings in the literature on successful aging. I hope you will find this crash course on optimal aging helpful.

Optimistic Aging

R esearch about aging has revealed an optimistic picture: the majority of older people feel well and live active, enjoyable lives. Furthermore, studies have shown that 70% of what is thought of as normal aging is preventable.[1] You read that right—70%! Lifestyle choices have much more of an impact on aging than most people realize.

The apparently inevitable effects of aging are actually a 30-year accumulation of unhealthy choices. Midlife is the ideal time to build healthy habits that will improve life now and set you up to be at your best with age. Even more promising are the findings that it's never too late to make healthy lifestyle choices to improve wellness.[2] Start taking better care of yourself now, no matter how many candles will be on next year's cake.

This book offers a concise summary of the research findings about aging well to inspire investment in your physical, mental, emotional, and social health. You will be able to have a vibrant life now, and for the duration.

When people think about growing old, they often focus on saving money for retirement. And while it is crucial to make sure that you have enough funds to support your lifestyle and medical needs, it is just as important to invest in all dimensions of health to age optimally and enjoy life fully.

70% of what is thought of as normal aging is preventable.

Financial planners urge us to start saving early so that our investments grow exponentially over time. Similarly, the sooner you invest in well-being, the more benefits you will enjoy. There is much to be done in your 40s, 50s, 60s, and beyond to remain vibrant in your 70s, 80s, and 90s. And unlike most retirement planning, wherein you must sock away money for it to grow into a nest egg for future use, wellness investments pay out right away. Nurture your physical, mental, emotional, and social health now to enrich your life in all those areas right away, as well as down the line.

Crash Course

This book provides a crash course about how to invest your time and energy wisely to have a healthier present and long-term future.

If you love to read and are interested in reading research summaries, this book may seem too sparse. You might want to read this as a primer or just skip to the recommended reading and notes sections for books and articles on the subject.

But for those of you who don't have the time or interest in reading in-depth research descriptions, this book is written with you in mind. I have studied the research and offer here a short and user-friendly summary of the key findings and recommendations.

This book can be read straight through, or by jumping to specific areas of concern. The first four chapters establish the mindset for change, developing your confidence, positive future vision, and action plan. The next four chapters address each of the four main focal areas of wellness: physical, mental, emotional, and social. The book closes with a discussion of how to put your plan into action.

It may inspire you to read this book cover to cover and see how many ways there are to make the future better. If you are likely to get overwhelmed, simply skim it to find something attainable and start there. Take as long as you need to solidify a new habit so it becomes automatic, then pick up the book again and choose a next step. Customize your path.

Interestingly, all four areas of health are heavily inter-related. For example, being physically active supports the maintenance of mental functioning, and vice versa. Any actions you take will likely support several areas of wellness.

Some action steps appear in more than one health area (for example, exercise is relevant to all four). I have written these sections with extra care to minimize redundancy, to keep you engaged, and to encourage further appreciation of each action step. Keep reading, even if it feels familiar.

Because of misinformation about aging, most people think they're on an inevitable downhill trajectory. However, much of what we fear about getting older is preventable.

To age optimally, you will need:

(1) knowledge about the right investments of your time and energy

(2) a mindset for change

(3) an effective plan to take action and stick with it

This book aims to help you in all of these areas.

The Choice Is Yours

Your choices now will affect your quantity and quality of life later. Your actions will impact your life in a healthy way, or in a way that leads to illness; therefore, it is important to have accurate information about how to promote current and future well-being. The health choices outlined in this book will make your life vibrant, regardless of its length, and will enable you to cope better with life's challenges, including illness and dying.

An interesting distinction in the aging literature is between having a diagnosed disease and feeling sick.[3]

Researchers observed that people struggling with chronic emotional or physical pain (alcoholism, depression, and arthritis) were more likely to feel sick regardless of their health status otherwise. On the other hand, they found many people with diagnosed diseases who did not experience themselves as ill subjectively. Even with medical problems, they felt well and lived vigorous lives. For example, my father was diagnosed with bladder cancer at age 30 and has worked closely with his doctors to successfully manage it for decades, all the while living a fulfilled life. Now he is 76 years old and still swims the butterfly stroke! When you are proactive about physical, mental, emotional, and social health, you will live and die feeling as well as possible.

Your choices now will affect your quantity and quality of life later.

Every day you make choices that greatly affect your quality of life for better or for worse. Don't forget that the default choice of inaction also has significant consequences. Use the information that follows to make educated decisions, focus your time and energy, and take charge of your life and future.

In the dance of life, you are the partner who leads. Your body takes its cues from your behavior and dances along in the chosen direction. Most people don't realize they are the lead dancer. They think they are at nature's mercy, with decline inevitable. But the research clearly shows that much of what we think of as aging decay is actually the result of lifestyle choices. This book will teach you the dance moves to effectively lead in the partnership with nature and twirl off into the sunset with flair. Once you know the moves, the choices are up to you.

2

Your Can-Do Spirit

To implement the health-promoting options contained in this book, you will need an action-able mindset. The most important component of this mindset is a sense of *self-efficacy*, which is psychobabble for personal optimism: the belief that your actions make a difference. Personal optimism empowers you to positively impact your life and the world and become willing to take action to improve your life.

The first and most critical step toward life-long vibrancy is to enhance your self-efficacy, your can-do spirit. Research clearly shows that this type of confidence is crucial to maintaining health and functioning with age.[1] A can-do spirit is essential to taking the action steps outlined in this book.

Start by thinking of the areas of life where you feel or have felt effective or impactful. For example, you might draw on professional or athletic accomplishments, or maybe your positive influence as a parent, spouse, or friend. Or this confidence could come from a hobby, wherein your hard work left you feeling pleased with your garden or proud of your piano performance.

Building your can-do spirit is essential to success in life and optimal aging.

Is it easy to find these experiences? If so, you probably have a strong can-do spirit already, and this will serve you well going forward.

If it is difficult to find areas where your actions have made a positive impact on your life, be assured that self-efficacy is like a muscle that can be strengthened, and make this your very first priority for aging well. Without a solid can-do spirit, the action steps in this book might seem out of reach, or worse, give you ammunition for self-blame. Take your time and get support to build self-efficacy. Building your can-do spirit is essential to success in life and optimal aging.

Everyone experiences disappointments—times when they feel unsuccessful or when their efforts result in negative outcomes. This is part of life. It is important to reflect upon setbacks to learn what you can from them. Once you have gleaned the wisdom offered by disappointing outcomes, it is crucial to redirect yourself to "Now what?" This will enable you to keep moving toward your goals and avoid getting bogged down in pessimism and low self-efficacy.

Another important aspect of resilience in the face of life's challenges is self-compassion. Notice how you speak to yourself when you make a mistake. Would you be this critical of loved ones? Is your self-talk supportive or condemning? If you tend to be unforgiving of your own shortcomings, try to be a better friend to yourself and speak more kindly internally. Self-compassion will enable you to try something new, be willing to make mistakes, and to get back up and keep going when you slip up.

Since a strong can-do spirit is the linchpin for successful aging, the first step of your journey is to develop a clear and solid experience of this self-efficacy.

For example, maybe you coached your daughter's basketball team to victory or felt the power of your empathy to soothe and reassure the girls when their team lost. Focus on the capacity of your mind to analyze and call the plays, the strength of your body to join in with the team's drills, and the warmth of your heart in helping the team regroup for a come-from-behind victory. Or maybe your successes have been professional. Savor the memory of your grace under pressure when you closed a difficult deal or made the right call in an emergency situation. Remember the tingling in your body as the intensity escalated and the calm of your mind as you quickly determined the right course of action. Or be warmed by your positive impact upon your relationships with friends, family, and community. Relive these experiences by remembering how you felt when people you care about responded positively to your efforts to connect with them. Soak up the warmth of imagining their ease in your presence, see them smiling at you, and recall their expressions of appreciation.

Consider the full scope of your life. What goals have required hard work? Where have your efforts had a positive impact? Breathe deeply and take several moments now to connect with what that confidence feels like. What other positive emotions surface? What thoughts come up while remembering these experiences of a can-do spirit? Scan your body from head to toe and notice what self-efficacy feels like. Savor those memories and let that confidence become as strong as it can. While remembering these positive experiences, make a mental highlight reel of this victory lap of successes.

The highlight reel is just that; it's meant to inspire and remind you that you can succeed. Even if it seems corny, practice your mental highlight reel on a regular basis, especially if you tend to be more pessimistic. Make sure the highlight reel is multifaceted and contains images, thoughts, feelings, and body sensations. This will help you connect with a vivid sense of self-efficacy, which provides the foundation upon which to build wellness. (For more about developing self-efficacy, see the Can-Do Spirit section of Chapter 7.)

My Highlight Reel

Take notes below about what came up in your highlight reel. Add to this list as new positive experiences occur.

I have had a positive impact in my life in these ways:

_____

_____

_____

_____

_____

_____

_____

_____

_____

_____

_____

_____

_____

_____

These positive thoughts, images, emotions, and body sensations arise when I think of my highlight reel:

_____

_____

_____

_____

_____

_____

_____

_____

_____

_____

_____

_____

_____

_____

_____

_____

3

A Vision for Your Vibrant Future

The second step in developing a mindset for change is to create a vision for your future that motivates you to make healthy choices.

Set aside any negative, preconceived notions about aging. Imagine a future where you might have slowed down a bit but can still function well physically and intellectually. In this vision, you are connected with family and friends, and you feel happy and fulfilled with life. Is it easy to envision this positive future? Can you think of older friends, family members, or public figures who are like this?

The ability to imagine yourself aging optimally is crucial to getting there.

Take the time to make your future vision as vivid as possible. Breathe deeply and imagine each dimension. Observe the images, thoughts, emotions, and physical sensations that arise as a visualization of your positive future develops. Take notes in the space provided at the end of the chapter to keep this vision handy while going forward.

The ability to imagine yourself aging optimally is crucial to getting there.

Imagine yourself physically decades from now, walking steadily and fluidly with upright posture. Picture yourself moving in whatever ways suit you. Will you be playing tennis, hiking, sightseeing in faraway destinations, or playing with your grandchildren? Regardless of how you feel now, experience the possibility that your body can be fit and strong. Let the awareness of your resilient body grow as strong as possible. Savor that experience while pausing to take notes at the end of this chapter about this visualization.

Think of remaining mentally stimulated and bright. Will you continue professional activities, learn a new language, volunteer at the local museum, or write a book? Regardless of how your mind feels now, know that if you choose to take action, your aging mind can be sharp and vibrant. You can have a high-functioning intellectual future. Let the awareness of your active mind become as strong as possible. Appreciate that experience while pausing to take notes about this vision.

Experience your heart feeling joyful and happy. Envision being able to deal with your own vulnerability graciously while maintaining confidence and excitement about life. Imagine the many things that will bring you joy: children, music, cooking, a good book, being out in nature. Make the list as long as possible. Regardless of how your mood feels at this time, experience the hope that your mood can be bright and your emotional skills formidable. You can have a joyful future. Let the awareness of your emotional vibrancy grow as strong as possible. Relish that experience while pausing to take notes.

Form a mental image of yourself years from now surrounded by a rich community of family and friends who value you. Imagine being connected with people of all ages with whom to share life's joys and sorrows. Picture comfortably receiving help when you need it, while also remaining as independent as desired. What social activities will you enjoy? Will it be traveling the world together, playing music with a group, skiing with others, or debating political ideas? Regardless of how connected you feel now, be optimistic and know that you can build a social circle of enjoyable and fulfilling relationships. Let the awareness of your connected self become as strong as it can. Savor that experience while pausing to take notes.

Now bring all of these aspects of your future together into an elaborate and vivid visualization. See yourself a little slower, a bit grayer, and with a few more wrinkles, but still physically active, mentally vivacious, cheerful, and connected with family and friends.

If you can find this without much struggle, you're on your way. If it is hard to imagine yourself with such a positive outcome, you might be overwhelmed by painful images of loved ones whose elderly experiences were nothing like this. Or maybe your current life is so far from this vision that it feels impossible to change your trajectory so dramatically. If it feels too impossible, then pick one area that is important or that feels the most accessible and imagine something more hopeful. You might also reflect on other people who are aging well and imagine yourself in their shoes, doing enjoyable activities. Start there and work on the other parts once you have experienced success in this first area.

Considering the vibrant future vision you just developed, keep in mind that these possibilities are available, though you will have to work to make them happen. The research is clear that lifestyle choices, more than genetics or life circumstances, are the key to aging successfully. As Harvard aging researcher Dr. George Vaillant concluded, "I was astonished at how much of a 70-year-old's healthy aging or lack thereof was predicted by factors already established before age 50. What seemed even more astonishing was that these factors are more or less controllable."[1]

The future vision created in this chapter will be a guide in prioritizing your efforts moving forward. Hopefully you are already on the right track in some areas, and the coming chapters will be reassuring. For the parts of your life that need more attention, you will find research-supported recommendations. Use this information to create a personal investment plan. Use your highlight reel to activate your can-do spirit and focus on the destination offered by your future vision. The remaining chapters will help you chart the course to get from here to there.

My Future Vision

Write a detailed description of your older, vibrant, and active self. Include positive outcomes for each area. Review this future vision regularly and revise it as your interests evolve over the years. Visualize this positive future frequently and tie it to your aging well plan.

Physical Health (mobility, activity, and feeling well)

Mental Functioning (intellectual interests, capacity)

Emotional Health (joyful, calm, resilient)

_____

_____

_____

_____

_____

_____

_____

_____

_____

_____

_____

_____

_____

_____

_____

_____

_____

_____

_____

_____

Social Health (community, connections)

_____

_____

_____

_____

_____

_____

_____

_____

_____

_____

_____

_____

_____

_____

_____

_____

_____

_____

_____

Getting There—One Step at a Time, For a Lifetime

You can only achieve your future vision one step at a time. The chapters that follow are filled with research-validated options for aging well. You cannot do all of these things right away, and some of the suggestions will never be a good fit for you. This book is intended to offer an à la carte menu of choices, not an all-you-can-eat buffet to overwhelm you.

Don't bite off more than you can chew. Start with a simple goal and move to more challenging tasks as your confidence grows. Prioritize your aging well plan based on your future vision and pick the components that are most important. Use any approach to get started, but be sure to do something.

To age well, whatever you choose needs to be a lifelong commitment. If lifestyle changes are to become permanent, they need to be manageable. You will need a specific plan to transform knowledge and good intentions into sustained action.

Working Against Your Autopilot

Changing bad habits is difficult because you are working against your brain and body. You are biologically designed, for maximum efficiency, to complete many actions without having to think about them. It is worth appreciating nature's brilliance when this automated function enables you to accomplish desirable habits with ease. But this biological autopilot system is hard to override when you are trying to change an unwanted habit or develop a new one.

> *Often, we are unaware of the chain of inner and outer events prompting our unwanted habits.*

Because much of daily living takes place in this automated, habitual mode, it is difficult to add something new or subtract an unwanted behavior. Imagine your daily routine as a train, with each car representing a specific behavior. The train has momentum and is moving down the track, making it difficult to remove a car or add a new one.

Habits are triggered by cues in the outer and inner environment. Preceding events, interactions with people, situational cues, thoughts, feelings, and temptations all work to flip the switch that activates automated behavior. Often, we are unaware of the chain of inner and outer events prompting our unwanted habits.

Awareness

Awareness is crucial for successful behavior change. In order to stop an unwanted habit or initiate a new one, you need to pay close attention to your thoughts, emotions, and behaviors, as well as the triggering situations (places and people). These observations provide information about the obstacles you are facing. These insights can then be used to develop intervention plans and identify cues for implementing these plans. All of this enables the shift from autopilot to the vigilant manual pilot to successfully change a habit.

When observing your inner experience, don't bother trying to suppress unwanted thoughts, feelings, and urges. The goal is simply to recognize these experiences and the triggers that cause them to arise. Research has shown that trying to suppress thoughts of unwanted habits just strengthens them.[1] Instead, observe the inner struggles and redirect yourself to the desired action. Habit expert Jeremy Dean noted that "successfully breaking a habit is much more likely when you have a shiny new, well-planned habit to focus on rather than just thinking about suppressing the old habit."[2]

The first new habit might need to be increasing awareness about the target issue. Begin by paying attention to your behavior, the situational cues that prompt your actions or inaction, and your thoughts and emotions. Ideally, take notes about these observations for a few weeks. For example, if you want to eat healthier, don't make any eating changes right away. Instead, take detailed notes on your relationship with food. This information will be very useful for developing an action plan, and this attentiveness will enable you to implement the plan and succeed in changing your eating behavior.

Make a Plan to Build a New Habit

Research about habit formation has shown that developing a specific action plan is essential for success. Once you select an action item, consider the issue in great detail and develop a series of "when–I will" plans.[3] For example, if you are trying to change your eating habits, you might specify, "When I have a snack, I will serve myself in a small bowl rather than eating directly out of the bag." The "when" components of these statements address the fact that habits are triggered by circumstances, and the "I will" statement initiates the new preferred behavior.

Set yourself up for success by anticipating the situational triggers for unwanted habits and using them as reminders to do something new. For example, people who are trying to quit smoking often chew gum because it gives them something else to reach for instead of a cigarette. It is most effective to replace an old habit with a new one, because it gives you something to step toward rather than just trying to resist temptation.

Making a specific plan is important because habits cannot be changed with willpower alone. Research has demonstrated that willpower is an exhaustible resource.[4] It is like a muscle in that it can be strengthened by successes, but it can also be worn out with too much strain. When faced with behavior decisions once your willpower is depleted, you will most likely default to old habits. Map out your "when–I will" plans while your willpower is strong and you are away from the triggers. By making the decisions ahead of time, it becomes easier to apply the new action, even when your willpower feels drained.

Another strategy for reinvigorating depleted willpower is to connect with core values.[5] When you recall what matters to you (e.g., relationships, creativity, beauty, your future vision), your mindset shifts and the temptation of the moment lessens, thus restoring self-control. It is crucial to have strategies like these to re-energize your efforts when willpower feels depleted.

Once a new habit is established, it is normal for old habits to creep back in. Use "when–I will" statements to anticipate these setbacks and get yourself back on course.

For example, "If I succumb to temptation and overeat, I will remind myself that it's normal to struggle with behavior change, and I will seek support to get back to my healthy eating plan."

WOOP It Up for Successful Change

One research-supported strategy for developing new habits is recalled by the acronym WOOP:[6]

Wish—What is the new habit you'd like to develop?
Outcome—What positive outcomes will this new habit create for your life?
Obstacles—What will make it difficult to develop the new habit (situations, people, emotions, thoughts, temptations)?
Plan—Specific action plans using "When–I will" statements to initiate the habit, help overcome obstacles, and get you back on track if derailed.

For example, here is a WOOP for a person who wants to eat better:

Wish—Healthy eating
Outcome—Reverse pre-diabetic status, have more energy, lose weight
Obstacles—Hunger, emotional eating, unconscious eating

<u>Plan</u>—I will carry nuts in my bag to have a healthy snack handy when I feel hungry. I will eat snacks throughout the day so I am less likely to experience hunger. When I'm upset, I will call a friend for support instead of eating. When I have a snack, I will eat with my non-dominant hand in order to pay more attention to how much I am eating.

The chapters that follow conclude with WOOP prompts, which are included to aid you in transforming intentions into lasting action.

Repetition

Once you have designed a plan of action for the new target behavior, you will need to commit to daily action. The key is repetition, repetition, repetition. The old habit may have had years of recurrences to solidify it as the dominant action. To break through that, your brain requires a period of regular repetition to weaken an old habit and/or rewire a new one.

By doing the new action daily for around two months, it will become wired into your body-memory and brain and become more automatic.

Studies about behavior change have shown that the average amount of time it takes to develop a new habit is about two months.[7] Some habits come more quickly; some take longer to establish. By doing the new action daily for around two months, it will become wired into your body-memory and brain and become more automatic. Once this happens, it's easier to keep it up for the rest of your life. Then you can choose to focus on another action item. (For a review of the research about habits, see Jeremy Dean's book, *Making Habits, Breaking Habits*.)

Make One Behavior Change at Time

Don't try to overhaul your lifestyle all at once. It is more effective to focus on making one behavior change at a time and do it really well. Since it takes approximately two months to establish a new habit, by the end of a year, you will have added as many as six new self-care actions. That's quite an accomplishment. And even if you stay with just one, you will be on a better life path than before. It's also important to note that many of the action options outlined in this book will influence multiple dimensions. For example, supportive relationships impact physical health, mental functioning, and mood. So instead of focusing on the quantity of changes, just pick something that will work for you, and stick with it.

Remember that once you do the hard work to plan and implement a change, it will be wired into your brain and body so that the autopilot will keep it going. When the new habit becomes routine, you can relax and enjoy the benefits of your effort.

There are numerous paths to follow to realize your future vision. It should be a slow and steady course—you have the rest of your life, after all. It's the lifelong commitment that truly matters the most. Though habit change is challenging, with the right approach, it can be done. Make a plan and stick with it, one step at a time.

Physical Health

We all aspire to high-quality longevity: a long, healthy, and happy life. We also want to die as painlessly as possible. Research on aging well shows that healthy lifestyle choices enable people to live vibrant, happy, and meaningful lives throughout their later years. Furthermore, the research shows that these lifestyle choices can improve dying as well.

Studies have shown that when death comes for successful agers, the period of disabling disease is relatively brief. The medical jargon for this is called *compression of morbidity*, which means shortening the disease period prior to death.[1] In some cases, people live disease-free until something finally takes them. For example, Joy Johnson died peacefully in her sleep the day after completing her 25th consecutive New York City Marathon at the age of 86![2] In other cases, people who have a medical disease don't feel ill and continue to enjoy a high quality of life.

In the stereotypical view of aging, the tipping point happens quickly and it's followed by a steady and difficult decline over many years prior to death. This is the pessimistic vision of aging: experiencing dementia and/or living bedridden for years before finally dying. My beloved grandmother spent her last five years wheelchair bound, helpless as an infant and suffering from Alzheimer's disease before her death at age 98. Unlike Joy, her morbidity was painfully prolonged, rather than compressed.

You can postpone and shorten your decline toward death by being proactive, and it is never too late to start.

Most people would postpone the tipping point toward death if given the choice. Medical advances have lengthened life, but they have not done much to improve the quality of life once decline sets in. Research has clearly identified the lifestyle choices that promote a high quality of life while aging. However, doctors can't change your lifestyle. You have to do that yourself.

It turns out that you actually have the choice to hasten or postpone the tipping point of your life. The bad news is that inaction results in a faster progression to the tipping point. Conversely, the choice to postpone the tipping point requires decisive self-care action for the rest of your life. You can postpone and shorten your decline toward death by being proactive, and it is never too late to start. Remember, you have the choice. What will you choose?

Exercise Regularly for the Rest of Your Life

Let's jump right in with a well-known fact: exercising is crucial to your health now and later. If you take away only one thing from this book, let it be the habit of exercise. Regular exercise, regardless of the intensity level, gives the biggest bang for the buck. There is nothing more important you can do for your long-term well-being than exercise.

Before continuing, I have to pause for a personal giggle about becoming an exercise advocate. I have been sedentary most of my life. Even knowing the benefits of exercise, I avoided it, eventually running out of excuses and then stalling for another year, repeating, "I just don't feel like it." Working on this project finally inspired action. I rallied my can-do spirit and applied it to regular physical activity. I won't bore you with my long list of hang-ups, but suffice it to say: if I can exercise, so can you. Exercise doesn't come naturally to me, but now I do it anyway because my future vision includes exploring the world and being physically active with my children and grandchildren.

The research about aging well is unanimous on the subject of exercise—use it or lose it. Both aerobic exercise and strength training are essential for optimal aging. As Chris Crowley and Dr. Harry Lodge, the authors of *Younger Next Year*, put it: "aerobic exercise saves your life and strength training makes it worth living."[3] Aerobic exercise is important for the prevention of the most lethal diseases: heart disease and stroke, as well as diabetes and some cancers. And strength training will keep you physically functional by preventing falls, broken bones, and arthritis. Recent research even shows that exercise affects you genetically: it influences the biochemical processes that turn on or off many of your genes (this process is called *epigenetics*). For example, one study found that genes involved in fat storage are impacted by exercise.[4]

The research about aging well is unanimous on the subject of exercise—use it or lose it. Both aerobic exercise and strength training are essential for optimal aging.

The research on aerobic exercise shows that it doesn't need to be vigorous to be effective, but consistency is a must. Dancing, walking, and even gardening will do the trick, as long as you do them regularly.

Aerobic exercise doesn't change the heart as much as it strengthens the circulatory system. Healthy circulation nourishes your muscles and organs by delivering oxygen and blood, but more importantly, circulation cleanses your entire system and decreases inflammation caused by inactivity.[5] While I'm exercising, I like to imagine the new capillaries forming throughout my body, creating an improved highway system for use by my internal catering service and HazMat team. Do something active every day for the rest of your life. Keep in mind that most of what people think of as the typical effects of aging are actually the effects of a sedentary lifestyle.

Be honest with yourself about your seated time (desk job, driving, reading, visiting with friends, computer time, etc.). If you aren't already, find some way to move daily. (For more on this, check out Dr. Mike Evans' YouTube video called "23 and 1/2 Hours: What is the Single Best Thing We Can Do for Our Health?") I started with a commitment to myself to go for a walk every day no matter what. This was where I made the startling discovery (which now seems obvious) that my legs were aching at the end of my long, seated workdays because they craved movement. For years, I put my feet up at the end of the day to rest my aching legs. Now I make time to exercise first thing in the morning when I see many hours of sitting on my calendar. I have also decreased my seated time by creating a standing desk in my office using an adjustable tray table on top of my desk (which I'm typing on now while standing).

The modern sedentary lifestyle confuses the primitive brain. Historically, the only reason to sit around rather than hunt or gather was because of famine. So the body interprets sitting—regardless of how much food we are chowing down—as a signal of scarcity. To cope with this perceived famine, the body switches into a physiological depression, which slows down all but the basic functions for survival. We hear about how our sedentary lifestyle causes obesity, but even more concerning is that inactivity signals the body to decay.[6]

Regular movement will turn off the decay signal. Even more exciting is the idea that we can give the body a growth signal by performing vigorous exercise. This isn't necessary for aging well (milder movement will do the trick), but if you want to feel truly vibrant, increase your exercise intensity. This will also help with weight management, as strenuous aerobic exercise and weight training increase your base metabolic rate; therefore, you will be burning calories even while sitting.[7]

The frequency, duration, and intensity of exercise matter. Consistent frequency is the most important of these, so whatever you choose, do it regularly. To send a growth signal, exercise with duration (30+ minutes) and intensity. If the goal is to turn down or turn off the decay signal, complete a longer, moderate workout such as a 30-minute walk or a shorter, intense workout. Research has shown that brief, intense exercise is as effective as longer, less-intense exercise.[8] Thus, if you don't have much time to fit in a workout, make it short and intense (for example, check out the *7 Minute Workout* app).

The definition of exercise intensity is based on what your heartbeat registers, not what your thoughts say. Before focusing on workout intensity, learn about optimal heart rates and how to use a heart monitor (Crowley and Lodge's *Younger Next Year* gives detailed instructions for the safe use of heart rate monitoring to increase intensity). If your heart says it's had enough, don't push past this.

IMPORTANT: Before starting any new exercise routine, be sure to get checked out by a doctor. Since the goal here is to help you live a long and vibrant life, it would be awful if you dropped dead because of an undetected heart condition or another undiagnosed ailment. Make sure to get your ticker checked out and obtain a thorough once-over while you're at it (more on this later). Also, consider starting with a personal trainer or physical therapist to avoid injury. Supervised and medically-endorsed exercise programs are safe, even for seniors.

It's equally important to build your fitness at the gym or with a physical therapist before undertaking demanding sports activities. Dr. Deb Saint-Phard, Director of the University of Colorado Women's Sports Medicine Clinic, urges her patients to "Get in shape to play. Don't play to get in shape."[9] She has seen many people who have been injured by jumping into a fun sports activity without enough prior exercise. So avoid blowing out your knee while skiing by strengthening your body before you hit the slopes.

Strength training, in addition to aerobic exercise, is essential for optimal aging. Lifting weights not only maintains and builds muscle, but it can treat or prevent arthritis and strengthen bones.

Strength training is also beneficial because it keeps the lines of communication open between the brain and body. Lifting weights sends a strong signal from the body to the brain to maintain the brain's awareness of the body in space (the medical jargon for this brain-body connection is *proprioception*). Older people don't stumble any more than younger people; however, they don't recover their balance as easily because of this communication breakdown.[10] Falls and brittle bones can lead to wheelchairs and a swift decline from which many don't recover.

Weightlifting can be intimidating. It certainly is for me. But there are lots of ways to get the job done. Ideally, as word continues to spread about how important weightlifting is for long-term health, the soft bodies will outnumber the hard bodies in the weightlifting section of the gym. Using free weights and weight machines are an important part of staying strong and high functioning. However, there are other approaches to build muscle. TRX workouts are a newer approach, while yoga has been around for centuries. It doesn't matter what you do, just do some type of strength training regularly to keep your bones and muscles strong.

Don't forget that your muscles need a spell to recover as they strengthen. Whereas it is safe to do aerobic exercise multiple days in a row, give your body a few days to rest and recover between weight-training sessions, allowing the muscle fibers time to rebuild before their next challenge.

Strength training gives us a life worth living. It aids in preventing and decreasing pain (arthritis), strengthening our bones (preventing osteoporosis), and maintaining our brain-body connection (proprioception).

It's never too late to start exercising. For example, in one study, residents in a nursing home, including many in their 90s, did a stint of weight training. In general, all participants improved: those who were bedridden moved to wheelchairs, those in wheelchairs moved to walkers or canes, and those using canes could walk without assistance.[11] By all means, start early to get that ounce of prevention, but if you are struggling with arthritis, talk with your doctor to determine if weight training is appropriate.

Another exciting finding is that exercise acts as an antidote to other risk factors. Research has shown that sedentary nonsmokers with normal blood pressure have a higher mortality rate than smokers or people with high blood pressure who exercise vigorously.[12] Even if you aren't quite ready to give up one or more of your vices, make sure to exercise to counteract the effects of your other risky choices.

There is much more to say about the benefits of exercise for aging well, but in the interest of keeping my promise to be concise, I will give a quick rave about the book *Younger Next Year* by Crowley and Lodge. This book will inspire you to move! With a playful and blunt tone, it provides an excellent explanation of the body's growth versus decay signal system, and it outlines how to crack the code to communicate growth signals to your body. This book transformed me from a couch potato to a runner. Granted, I'm a slow runner (both of my children can lap me in a 5K), but I'm still a runner, thanks to *Younger Next Year*, and I can feel the benefits in my physical, mental, and emotional health.

Don't Go on a Diet

Weight management is a loaded topic for most people who have attempted and failed to lose weight. You may have given up trying. If this is true for you, then start somewhere else and come back to this challenge once your can-do spirit feels stronger.

While maintaining a healthy weight is important for aging well, being thin can be dangerous. With regard to aging, thin can equal frailty, which is a risk factor for poor health. If you have been wrestling with a few extra pounds, relax and appreciate that bit of padding as protection.

If you carry more than a few extra pounds, dieting should still be avoided. Overall, diets don't work for the long haul. They yo-yo body weight around and leave you feeling depleted and discouraged. A recent study showed that extreme dieting left participants in a biologically altered, starvation-like state a full year after significant weight loss, even after the pounds returned.[13]

If you struggle with obesity, focus on self-compassion as your first action step. The book *The Self-Compassion Diet* by Jean Fain is an excellent resource for building the emotional foundation and awareness needed for successful behavior change. Self-criticism will make any action steps about exercise or eating differently very difficult. Furthermore, research has shown that the risk for obesity is genetic.[14] As a result, reaching and staying at a healthy weight may be harder, though it is still possible. Remember, your can-do spirit is your most important resource, and it can be difficult to connect with this confidence if you are feeling criticized and discouraged.

In addition to treating yourself compassionately, seek support from people who understand how difficult these challenges are and who won't be judgmental. The equivalent of a personal trainer for food is a nutritionist who can improve your food awareness and help with meal planning.

Also, a therapist can help you develop a healthier relationship with food. Weight Watchers provides social support to participants, and Overeaters Anonymous is a free support group based on the AA model. Look for help to develop healthy eating habits for the rest of your life.

Once you are ready to address food intake, keep in mind that from a nutritional perspective, it is important to eat well and practice portion control. There are countless nutrition books, and they include conflicting advice about what foods are healthy to eat. My favorite nutrition advice is from Crowley and Lodge: "Stop eating crap."[15] It's the crap that clogs up the works and threatens your health.

Begin by eliminating one unhealthy item from your diet at a time. Try living without potato chips or donuts for two months, for example. Or switch from red meat to chicken or fish. Pick something doable. Make a two-month commitment, because you will likely feel worse before feeling better. Junk food is designed by the food industry to create cravings, so you will probably miss the chips and sodas for a while before the benefits of avoiding unhealthy items kick in.

If you already avoid junk food, you might want to focus on adding healthier foods. Almost everyone can benefit from adding more veggies. Ideally, more than half of your plate should include a colorful array of vegetables. Learn how to cook them in ways that you enjoy. In order to make eating healthier a lifelong habit, food needs to taste good to motivate you to continue eating healthy food for the duration.

It is also important to focus on what and how much you drink. Dehydration is common and causes significant health problems, including dizziness, cognitive confusion, and loss of balance, so staying hydrated is important. There is a greater risk of dehydration with age because the sensation of thirst decreases due to declining kidney function.[16] This means that you may become dehydrated without your body signaling you to drink more. Don't wait for your body to say it's thirsty. Drink non-caffeinated, nonalcoholic beverages regularly throughout the day. It doesn't always have to be water; just stay hydrated.

In addition to healthy food choices, another helpful option for weight management is to decrease food intake. Your base metabolic rate slows as you age, so you'll need less fuel to keep the engine running at the same speed.[17] One way to increase awareness of healthy portion size is to use a smaller plate for meals. When eating out, eat half of the portion and take the other half home for the next day. Eating healthy snacks in between smaller meals can also help with weight management.

You might be surprised to learn that getting more sleep can also help you manage your weight. Recent research has discovered a "neuroendocrine cascade" that links sleep deprivation to obesity.[18] If you aren't getting seven to eight hours of sleep per night, consider going to bed earlier to support your body's metabolism. Ironically, this sedentary behavior is as important to health and weight management efforts as being physically active. (For more information about improving sleep habits, see the Prioritize Sleep section in Chapter 6.)

Whatever weight management strategy you embrace, make it doable so that it becomes a lifelong habit. Again, avoid extreme diets, because they are not sustainable and just leave you feeling deprived.

Keep Your Friends Close and Your Family Closer

Staying connected is good for your health. People who are involved in community are physically healthier, and they live longer than those who are isolated.[19]

Marriage and other family relationships, faith-group involvement, friendships, and community participation are sources of social fulfillment that protect physical health as you age. Relationships with pets can also provide social connection. It is not important that you are a social butterfly, but, rather, that you have a solid social network to experience the power of connection.

Research about social support's impact on physical health shows that the secret sauce is the emotional support we receive from and give to those with whom we are connected. Interestingly, hands-on help with tasks is not necessarily beneficial to elderly people. It can be detrimental to physical functioning and the can-do spirit when people stop doing things they could have done for themselves. What improves physical (mental and emotional) functioning is being heard, supported, cared about, and encouraged by others.[20]

Earlier I said to develop only one new habit at a time; however, strengthening your social support system is one place to get a twofer. Consider implementing one of your new habits in a social setting. For example, you can meet people with similar interests by taking a class. This way you strengthen your social support network while stretching your brain, and all of this keeps your body healthier. That's a win-win-win!

Stop Smoking and Abusing Alcohol

You already know that smoking and alcoholism cause premature death, so I won't belabor those findings. The research is also clear that smoking and abusing alcohol are the strongest predictors of those who are sad and sick in their old age.[21]

Both smoking and alcohol abuse are physiological addictions. While it is important to stop smoking and manage alcoholism, it is very difficult to do. People who haven't experienced these addictions don't know what it is like to break free of the physiological and mental grip of cravings. The struggle associated with these behaviors is exacerbated by the societal judgments about smoking and alcoholism.

The research is clear that smoking and abusing alcohol are the strongest predictors of those who are sad and sick in their old age.

If you smoke, you know that cigarettes are a stimulant. For many, smoking is a habit and not a conscious decision. In order to quit, you will need support and strategies to redirect yourself when tempted to smoke. Reach out for support from other people who have stopped smoking, because they understand the difficulties involved with quitting, or call 1-800-QUIT-NOW for free professional support. Talk with your doctor about smoking cessation medications. The most effective approach is a combination of counseling and medication. You can do this, and you are not alone. As of 2002, there were more former smokers than current smokers in the US.[22]

If quitting smoking feels too difficult, then make it a priority to add an aerobic exercise program. You can mitigate some of the harm of smoking by strengthening your lungs through aerobic activity.[23] Hopefully, in time you'll quit smoking and make exercise a priority, but at least do one for now.

The great news is that stopping smoking has immediate medical benefits, and it is never too late to make a positive health difference by quitting. The risk of heart disease decreases almost immediately after smoking cessation. In two to four years, those who quit smoking before age 55 were at no more risk of a stroke than those who had never smoked. The same is true for heart disease after stopping for five years. In 15 years, the risk of lung cancer is the same as for those who never smoked. Every day you don't smoke, your body gets stronger and your health recovers.

While there is clear consensus that smoking is dangerous for your health, society's views about alcohol are more complex. Most American adults drink alcohol to some extent, and some studies even suggest that a drink a day will keep the doctor away. However, the research is clear that alcohol addiction is a significant risk factor for illness and often leads to premature death.

How can you tell the difference between alcoholism and benign alcohol use? One key distinction is that alcoholics feel a strong compulsion to drink, and they have difficulty limiting the amount of alcohol they consume. In addition, alcoholics develop a tolerance and thus require more and more alcohol to experience the same desired level of intoxication. When deprived of alcohol, addicts suffer from physiological withdrawal symptoms (shaking, nausea, perspiring). Alcoholics may also experience blackouts, where they don't remember what they did during a drunken episode.

It is difficult, though not impossible, to address alcoholism without professional treatment or a peer support group. Because of withdrawal symptoms, hospitalization is sometimes required to medically monitor the transition from using to sobriety. After detoxification, it is crucial to develop an action plan to identify triggers and build alternative skills to cope with stressors. Medications are also available to help eliminate cravings or the perceived good feelings that come with alcohol use. Ongoing support is very important for successful treatment of alcohol abuse.

You may not know that alcohol is a depressant. It physiologically depresses mood and body functions. This is ironic, because people often turn to alcohol in an attempt to alleviate distress. However, prospective studies (meaning that people are studied over decades as their lives unfold) of adult development have shown that the life stressors come after, not before, the excessive drinking started.[24] Alcohol abuse causes increased stress, depression, relationship problems, and downward social mobility. A vicious cycle ensues, because people feel the need for alcohol to cope with their despair, often not realizing that their "comfort in a bottle" is the cause of their distressing circumstances.

If you see the signs of alcoholism in yourself, it is probably daunting to think about addressing this issue.

Alcohol often poses as a consoling friend, promising to make you feel better. And it succeeds—at first. Because of alcohol's seductive effects, it is often hard to keep in mind the long-term consequences of abuse when the next moment feels intolerable without a little something to take the edge off.

Alcoholics often struggle with shame. If friends and family are critical of your drinking, it might be hard to consider this issue without feeling defensive. Keep in mind that addiction is genetic. While you can't change this genetic vulnerability, you can stop the behavior of alcohol abuse. Cultivate self-compassion and seek support. Breaking free of the physical dependency, mental obsessiveness, and anguish of alcoholism is difficult, but possible. You can manage alcoholism, and you will live longer and have a better quality of life sober.

Treat Depression

A history of depression correlates with an increased likelihood of coronary heart disease and Alzheimer's disease.[25] Depression and arthritis cause people's subjective experience of their health to be worse than those without these forms of chronic pain.[26] Finally, depression kills the can-do spirit, which may be its greatest threat to aging well. Self-efficacy is the cornerstone to healthy aging, and depression introduces self-defeating and pessimistic thinking, which leaves people feeling discouraged about taking action to care for themselves and their future.

Clinical depression is distinct from the normal experience of having a down day or two and from the experience of bereavement after a loss. A depressive episode involves depressed or irritable mood or a loss of interest in your usual daily activities for two or more weeks. In addition, clinical depression involves an increase or decrease of appetite, weight, and/or sleep; energy depletion; feelings of guilt or worthlessness; concentration problems; and/or suicidal thinking. Depression can be unipolar (only depression) or bipolar (depression alternating with mania or hypomania, which involve abnormally elevated mood and other symptoms).

If you struggle with depression, you might feel weak or think you have a character flaw. Depression is a biological disease that manifests in mood, cognitive, and/or behavioral symptoms. You haven't caused the problem, it just happens; however, the solution is up to you.

Depressive disorders are treatable. Research has shown that depression is responsive to cognitive-behavioral psychotherapy interventions, such as Acceptance Commitment Therapy (known as ACT). Treatment with medication is also effective for bringing depression into remission.

If you are struggling with depression, reach out for help. Talk with your family, friends, or your doctor. Find a therapist or read an ACT self-help book (such as *The Mindfulness and Acceptance Workbook for Depression* by Strosahl and Robinson). Address depression soon, because everything else will be easier to do once you feel better and recover your can-do spirit.

Visit Your Doctor; Take this To-Do List with You

If you think that doctors are only helpful for illness, you are missing a crucial opportunity for optimal aging. Work with your doctor proactively to identify and treat warning signs before problems arise.

The MacArthur Foundation funded an interdisciplinary research team to conduct extensive studies on successful aging over an eight-year period. The MacArthur researchers identified a group of symptoms that typically are considered normal effects of aging, but actually are early warning signs of disease. Their adamant recommendation is to watch these indicators closely and treat them once they start to creep up, before they cross the line to disease.

The MacArthur researchers identified a group of symptoms that typically are considered normal effects of aging, but actually are early warning signs of disease.

The MacArthur Study called this cluster of symptoms Syndrome X and showed that these symptoms eventually lead to diseases, including some cancers, and even more often, strokes and heart attacks.[27] Work with your doctor to track the following indicators:

- Body weight increase, especially abdominal fat
- Blood pressure increase, including just systolic (the top number)
- Blood fat increase (such as cholesterol and triglycerides)
- Blood sugar and insulin level increases
- Immune function decrease
- Bone density and muscle mass losses
- Lung function decrease (If you become winded easily, request measurement of your pulmonary peak expiratory flow rate; it is one of the best predictors of how much longer you will live, and lung function can be strengthened with aerobic exercise.)

Changes in these indicators are common in midlife, and these symptoms can be modified *before* they become disease. Some doctors might prefer to wait until these symptoms have crossed the threshold for disease. If this is true of your doctor, advocate for yourself and point to the MacArthur Foundation research and recommendations.

Weight loss is the most important intervention to control Syndrome X. Most of these symptoms are outcomes of a sedentary lifestyle. Exercise is crucial for preventing these symptoms in the first place, and it can help in treating Syndrome X. Medication for increased blood pressure is safe, inexpensive, and effective for preventing hypertension, especially if your systolic blood pressure (the top number) is over 160, and, in some cases, above 140. Talk with your doctor if this applies to you (and consult the AHA/ACC/CDC Science Advisory regarding high blood pressure control[28]).

Regular exams with your doctor can provide early detection of cancer. You might avoid your doctor because just imagining him/her reaching for the rubber gloves makes you want to run in the other direction! While certain exams may be uncomfortable, they are much less intrusive and difficult than cancer treatment. Make an appointment for that dreaded rectal and colon exam, skin exam, mammogram, pelvic exam, and Pap smear. Early intervention is crucial for surviving cancer and thriving thereafter. (For more on this, check out the American Cancer Society's "Guidelines for the Early Detection of Cancer."[29])

Hormone supplementation is a controversial subject in aging research and the findings on this issue are too contradictory to make any recommendations here. If you are considering hormone replacement therapy for menopause or andropause (male hormonal changes), please look closely at the debates and discuss this subject at length with your doctor before making a decision.

Once you are over 65, get an annual flu shot and pneumococcal vaccine, as well as a tetanus vaccination or booster.

Finally, it is important to know your health risk profile. While 70% of physical aging is related to lifestyle, genetics play a greater role in premature death.[30] If you have family members who died young, work closely with your doctor to be proactive. See your doctor regularly, keep an eye on disease warning signs, and intervene aggressively if they start creeping up.

Wear Sunscreen

Most anti-aging interventions focus on appearance. Our culture values the appearance of youth; therefore, we have booming cosmetic surgery and anti-aging industries to help people avoid looking old. While they haven't yet figured out how to keep hair from graying and thinning, it is clear how to prevent wrinkles.

What you think of as the effects of aging on skin is actually caused by sun exposure.[31] The best way to preserve your youthful appearance is to avoid intense sun exposure and wear sunscreen with a minimum SPF of 15 every day.

Cover all exposed skin areas, and don't forget to apply it to the backs of your hands. Reapply if you are outside for more than two hours and after swimming or getting sweaty. Seek shade midday and wear lightweight clothing, sunglasses, and hats to cover up.

Even more important than preventing wrinkles, sun protection helps to prevent skin cancer. The most common form of cancer in the US, skin cancer is most often caused by ultraviolet (UV) radiation from sun exposure. Reduce the risk of getting skin cancer by wearing sunscreen and covering up. Your skin is the largest organ of your body, and it needs protection. This simple intervention offers a big benefit for your health.

What Will You Choose?

In reflecting on what you've just read about how to support your physical health, consider where you might start (or continue if you are already doing many of these things). What will you choose for your first action target? What can you realistically do for two months to establish a new lifelong habit? Use the worksheets on the following pages to develop an action plan.

My Physical Health Action Plan

Review the action options for strengthening your physical health. Use this list to develop a customized action plan. Put a check in front of any item you are already doing and an X next to any not relevant to you. Number the remaining items in order of how easily they can be integrated into your daily life. Or, you might rank order them in terms of how important they are to you.

_____ Regular aerobic exercise

_____ Regular strength training

_____ Make healthier food choices

_____ Stay hydrated

_____ Take smaller portions

_____ Expand / deepen my relationships

_____ Stop smoking

_____ Stop abusing alcohol

_____ Treat depression

_____ Work with my doctor to avoid Syndrome X and detect cancer early

_____ Wear sunscreen

Pick one physical health action item and write it here:

Before developing your WOOP, use your awareness about this action item to write detailed observations about your current behaviors, urges, thoughts, and feelings, as well as the situational triggers associated with any unwanted behaviors:

Use your observations to develop your WOOP for this physical health action item.

Wish—What is the new habit you'd like to develop?

_____

_____

_____

_____

_____

_____

_____

_____

_____

_____

_____

_____

_____

_____

_____

_____

Outcome—What positive outcomes will this new habit create for your life?

_____

_____

_____

_____

_____

_____

_____

_____

_____

_____

_____

_____

_____

_____

_____

_____

_____

_____

Obstacles—What will make it difficult for you to develop the new habit (situations, people, emotions, thoughts, temptations)?

_____

_____

_____

_____

_____

_____

_____

_____

_____

_____

_____

_____

_____

_____

_____

Plan—Develop specific action plans using "When–I will" statements to initiate the habit, successfully overcome obstacles, and/or get back on track if derailed.

6

Mental Functioning

The research on mental functioning with age also offers an optimistic perspective. While some areas of cognitive ability decline with age, the mental functioning required for independent living and intellectual engagement is generally not impacted by age. About 10% of people between the ages of 65–100 have Alzheimer's disease, with the most disruptive cognitive losses happening very late in life. The vast majority of elderly people retain their cognitive abilities while they continue to work and contribute.

Mental functioning associated with age is also heavily impacted by lifestyle choices. The MacArthur Study found three key variables that predicted strong cognitive ability in old age: regular physical activity, strong social support, and high self-efficacy (can-do spirit).[1]

A new understanding of the brain's resiliency is one of the most exciting scientific discoveries in recent years. The old beliefs were that we have a limited number of brain cells and that established neural networks could not be modified.

This way of thinking suggested the aging brain could only deteriorate and new learning was difficult. Brain imaging technology dispels this idea and illuminates a different understanding of how the brain works. We now know that the brain is flexible and resilient. Scientists refer to the brain's malleability as *neural-plasticity*, and *neurogenesis* is the growth of new brain cells. This paradigm shift offers great hope for your aging brain.

The brain has about 86 billion neurons. Think about that! That's a lot of raw material to harness. Individual neurons connect with each other as mental and behavioral functions develop. These connections are referred to as *neural networks*. I imagine them like constellations in the sky; only, in this case, the neurons reach for each other and impact one another via chemicals called *neurotransmitters*. Psychologist Donald Hebb observed that "neurons that fire together, wire together" to form neural networks.[2] The most important thing to know about your brain is that your choices of thought and behavior determine how these networks form. While it is harder to change neural networks as you get older, research has shown that the brain continues to be malleable into old age.

You have many options to retain—and even improve—your mental functioning as you age. While you review the research findings and recommendations that follow, think about which action items are a good fit for you and where you can get started.

Exercise for Brain Health

Regular aerobic exercise is the most important activity for reviving or maintaining your mental functioning.[3] Aerobic activity supports the circulatory system, which delivers fuel and clears waste throughout the body and brain. In addition to increasing the blood volume in the brain, exercise also stimulates nerve growth factor. This chemical protects existing brain cells and encourages them to connect, at the same time promoting neurogenesis: the growth of new brain cells.

Studies have shown that a sedentary lifestyle results in cognitive sluggishness. The addition of regular aerobic activity will sharpen your mind and improve *fluid intelligence*, the capacity for quick, creative thinking.[4] Furthermore, cardio exercise dramatically lowers your risk for Alzheimer's disease and other forms of dementia, as well as stroke, which can be cognitively debilitating. (For more about the benefits of exercise on the brain, see John Medina's book *Brain Rules*.)

Make regular aerobic activities a priority. For example, take a walk during your lunch break to function more effectively once you are back at work. Or consider a treadmill desk. Much of this book was researched and written on a treadmill desk. Though I'm walking slowly while working, I'm moving rather than sitting, thus decreasing my sedentary time.

Teach Yourself Something New

Regardless of your level of formal education, it is critical to keep your mind active. Your intellect craves stimulation; the more your intellect is engaged, the more cognitive abilities you will retain, which results in a desire to seek further stimulation. This virtuous cycle will propel you forward.

Brain neurons have *dendrites* that act like arms, reaching toward other neurons to form neural networks. When you engage in habitual activities, neural networks that have already formed continue to fire. While it is good to keep your usual routines in place, the best way to give your brain a workout is to do something new. This means that if you have always played the piano, continuing won't stimulate your brain to the extent it would for someone who is beginning to play. Learning something new causes the arms of your neurons (dendrites) to move and stretch into new directions toward other cells. This type of brain workout keeps the brain flexible and strong.

One of the things that will change with age is learning speed. It is important to seek learning circumstances where you can set your own pace, avoid distraction, and have opportunities for practice. Pick something new, don't rush, and practice, practice, practice.

The new learning you choose doesn't have to be an intellectual pursuit. Any new activity will stretch your brain. Take up yoga, become a better listener, or even brush your teeth with your non-dominant hand—anything new will do the trick. When you practice a new skill, your brain has to work, and a challenge keeps your brain healthy.

Another strategy for stretching brain neurons is to consider alternative viewpoints. Think about your entrenched beliefs and be your own devil's advocate. Can you find the holes in your own views, or the strengths of a different perspective? Consider an area of conflict with a friend or family member and try to understand the opposing point of view. This will increase your mental flexibility, and it will strengthen your relationships too.

Your brain will be strengthened by any actions that are different from your typical habits. All new wellness activities are, by definition, exercises for your brain. Even if you focus on physical fitness or improving relationships, your brain will stretch. How's that for a win-win?

Address Cognitive Decline with Brain Training

Another option for stretching your brain involves doing mental exercises to strengthen faltering cognitive skills. Research has shown that specific brain exercises can reverse memory loss and improve mental functioning. The MacArthur Study found that with training, older people did better on cognitive tasks than younger people without training.[5] It's encouraging to know you can get your cognitive mojo back.

Most brain training activities involve computer programs or smartphone apps that present various tasks to exercise brain circuits. Learning targets include memory, processing speed, sustaining attention, reasoning, and problem-solving abilities. The programs take you through a series of tasks and provide feedback about your progress. While the tasks may be difficult at first, with practice, you will see improvement. These tasks will stretch your brain, rebuild faulty connections, and create new ones.

> **With mental training and other brain stimulating activities, your cognitive skills will be expanded.**

The most widely known brain training program is Lumosity (www.lumosity.com). There are other options, including Brain Age (Concentration Training, Nintendo), HAPPYneuron (www.happy-neuron.com), and CogniFit (www.cognifit.com). You can also devise your own cognitive exercises, including the old-fashioned matching game using a deck of cards turned face down on the table. The key is bringing your full attention and effort to the task at hand. Challenge your memorization skills at a cocktail party (but skip the cocktails) by learning and practicing people's names as they are introduced and throughout the evening.

For the greatest impact, pick training experiences that are meaningful to you. Your brain shrinks with age, selectively pruning away neural connections to remain functional.[6] This mental downsizing means that you can't store it all, so work on what is most important to you. With mental training and other brain stimulating activities, your cognitive skills will be expanded. Don't fill yourself up with junk—pick things that matter.

Don't Retire

The dictionary offers the following synonyms for retire: withdraw, retreat, pull back, disengage, go away, shut oneself away (ouch!). By all means, don't retire. Stay engaged in your life. That might be by continuing at your job, or it might involve stimulating, unpaid activities.

If your job is enjoyable and provides intellectual stimulation, stick with it as long as you want. Many older people continue to succeed in paid work settings, or they shift to a volunteer role in their chosen field. Working will stimulate your mind and maintain your physical health and mental functioning.

Most people leave their paid job because the flexibility they desire isn't available, or because they have become physically disabled. Keep your health strong so that your employment ends when you decide it should, and not because of health problems.

Once you finish with paid work, seek situations that encourage mental stimulation. Even better, develop other interests prior to leaving work so you feel excited about retiring when the time feels right. What are your interests and hobbies? Do you want to learn a foreign language or learn to play a musical instrument? How about delving into gardening, cooking, art, community theater, or chemistry? What will keep your mind engaged?

Follow the excellent advice of one of the successful agers in the MacArthur Study: "Always maintain more interests than there's time for."[7] The average time from retirement to death is 15 years (an increase from an average of just three years of retirement over a century ago). To ensure those years are meaningful, become a collector of interests and activities. Avoid inactivity in retirement and go for active engagement instead, so that when you withdraw from work, it is because you are "going for it" in a new direction.

Further Your Education

Research consistently reports that people who have more years of education retain their cognitive abilities better, are physically healthier, and live longer.[8] The mental stimulation of formal education stretches the brain's neural connections. In addition, those with more education are likely to be drawn to intellectual leisure activities (reading, chess, playing an instrument, etc.), which further stretch their brains.

One hypothesis suggests that higher education provides access to jobs that increase intellectual flexibility. Employment that requires education may offer more opportunities for independent problem solving and cognitive challenges, as compared to jobs where you are closely supervised and directed by someone else. Challenges at work can positively impact your can-do spirit and the ability to retain mental functioning with age.

How is your mind stimulated? If your job doesn't engage your intellect much, how else could your thinker be activated?

Even without pursuing a degree, you can still take interesting classes. Look for continuing education opportunities at the local university, college, and community college. Attend lectures at the local library or bookstore. Explore the wealth of learning opportunities available via technology. For example, find interesting TED Talks online (www.ted.com/topics); explore podcasts and turn your commute into an educational experience; discover Khan Academy for brief lessons on countless subjects (www.khanacademy.org); go to Coursera (www.coursera.org) and take an online class from professors at America's top universities; or read blogs, books, or magazines on an intriguing subject.

We live in an era where you can educate yourself at your convenience, for free or inexpensively. There are endless ways to get a great brain workout.

Your brain is the conductor of the train that is your body. Keep the train conductor alert and healthy so the train doesn't derail.

Protect Your Head

Head injuries and concussions can lead to decreased mental functioning. A vehicle crash is the most likely cause of head trauma, so wear your seatbelt. If you enjoy exercise that puts your head at risk (cycling, skiing, horseback riding, etc.), be sure to wear a helmet. Even if you are a skilled driver and skier, others might not be, so protect your noggin.

If you have suffered previous concussions, you are at greater risk for mental deterioration, and it's even more important that your head is protected. Nurture and strengthen your brain, especially if it has been injured.

Focus on Folate

Research on Alzheimer's disease has shown a link between folate deficiency and brain atrophy (deterioration).[9] Folate exists in many foods, including liver, poultry, pork, green leafy veggies, asparagus, brussels sprouts, avocados, beans, and nuts. Folic acid is the synthetic form of folate used to fortify foods and offered in supplement form. Pastas, breads, and cereals are often fortified with folic acid.

Causes of folate deficiency include poor diet, excessive alcohol intake, diseases (e.g., celiac and Crohn's disease), genetic mutation (e.g., MTHFR), and medication interactions. Folate deficiency can cause high homocysteine levels, which put you at greater risk for Alzheimer's disease as well as blood clots, stroke, heart disease, and hypertension.

Increase your folate consumption by making dietary changes to include more folate-rich foods. Also be aware that a food's folate content can be lost by overcooking. Steaming veggies helps retain their folate. If you decide to take a folic acid supplement, talk with your doctor first. Vitamin B12 and B6 deficiencies, common in older adults, can be masked with folic acid supplementation, so get your vitamin B levels checked first.[10]

Prioritize Sleep

Although sleep seems like a dormant resting period, the brain is more active during 80% of sleep than when we are awake. While you slumber, your brain is busy *consolidating* the day's experiences and learning.[11]

Sleep needs and patterns vary considerably from person to person. The general recommendation is to sleep seven to eight hours per night, but some people need more or less. True for all of us is that *sleep debt* impacts mental, emotional, and physical functioning. When we aren't sleeping enough, it's harder to sustain attention, plan, and execute tasks; remember things and solve problems. Mood suffers, and with severe sleep deprivation, the body stops moving as commanded when performing fine and gross motor tasks. To be at your best mentally (not to mention emotionally and physically), make sleep a priority. (For more on how sleep works and impacts mental functioning, see *Brain Rules* by John Medina.)

If you aren't getting the recommended seven to eight hours of sleep per night (or whatever is your ideal), why is that? Are you staying up late working, watching TV, or reading? Or do you suffer from insomnia?

Getting enough sleep will help you think more clearly, be more efficient, and manage your weight.

For those of you who are able to sleep but are staying up late or getting up too early, remember that your body is performing essential tasks while sleeping, and commit to adjusting your sleep schedule. Start winding down earlier or set the alarm later. Getting enough sleep will help you think more clearly, be more efficient, and manage your weight (for more on this, see Chapter 5, Don't Diet).

If you struggle with insomnia, try adding structure by going to sleep and waking at consistent times every day, including weekends. Avoid electronic screens (TVs, computers, cell phones) an hour before bedtime, and keep the bedroom dark. Your bed should be a place for sleeping, not tossing and turning. If you wake up in the night and cannot fall asleep after a few minutes, get out of bed and do something else (without electronic screens) for a while to unwind. Exercise during the day can help, but the research shows that it takes several months for exercise to improve sleep.[12]

Connect in Conversation

Research on cognitive functioning shows that people with social connections have higher mental functioning than people without.[13] As with physical health, the key is to establish emotionally supportive relationships rather than receiving hands-on assistance. For brain health, engaging conversations are particularly important—the deeper and more meaningful, the better.

Showing up for a class about a subject of interest is good, but it's even better to have a conversation with someone about it afterward. Your neurons' dendrites (arms) will stretch more when you summarize what was learned, share your opinions, and think about what others have to say. A better brain workout happens when you consider the views and reactions of other people, especially if they are different from yours.

Pay attention to both listening and contributing to the conversation. Rich conversations have healthy back-and-forth dialogue. Pipe up if you tend to be reserved; or conversely, if you usually dominate conversation, focus on listening. If the conversation stalls and you aren't sure how to get it moving again, find a question to draw out your companion. Listening and being heard are the main ingredients of supportive relationships.

Stroke Prevention Is Alzheimer's Disease Prevention

Many of the findings summarized in this chapter come from a groundbreaking study by epidemiologist Dr. David Snowdon. He and a team of researchers studied 678 nuns, aged 75 to 106, throughout their later years, including a study of their brains after death. These women contributed much to our understanding of cognitive functioning with regard to aging and Alzheimer's disease.

Alzheimer's disease is assessed in life but formally diagnosed after death, when a brain autopsy may reveal the telltale signs of Alzheimer's disease: tangles and plaques in the brain, and brain shrinkage. In his research, Snowdon was surprised to find that some nuns who functioned well during cognitive assessments just prior to death had severe tangles and plaques in their brains, as well as brain shrinkage. This startling finding demonstrates that one can have the brain manifestations of Alzheimer's disease without experiencing the cognitive decline of dementia.

Brain attacks seem to act as a trip switch for Alzheimer's disease in that, if you have a vulnerability to the disease, having a stroke may cause the otherwise dormant cognitive symptoms of Alzheimer's disease to emerge.

As Dr. Snowdon went on to explore the differences between those who manifested Alzheimer's symptoms and those who didn't—even when their brains showed impact—stroke became a clear culprit.[14] Another term for a stroke is a brain attack. When a blood clot occurs in the heart, it's referred to as a heart attack; a stroke is a blood clot in the brain. Brain attacks seem to act as a trip switch for Alzheimer's disease in that if you have a vulnerability to the disease, having a stroke may cause the otherwise dormant cognitive symptoms of Alzheimer's disease to emerge.

The good news is while we don't know much about how to prevent Alzheimer's disease yet, we do know a great deal about stroke prevention. The keys to preventing stroke include treating high blood pressure, heart disease (especially atrial fibrillation), high cholesterol and diabetes, smoking cessation, and addressing alcohol abuse. Folate deficiency and homocysteine elevations are implicated in strokes as well, which might explain their connection to Alzheimer's disease. If you have concerns about being vulnerable to Alzheimer's disease, redouble your efforts to avoid having a stroke by addressing the issues previously listed through exercise and weight loss. (For more information on stroke prevention, see www.stroke.org.)

What Will You Choose?

In reflecting on what you've just read about how to support your mental functioning, consider where you might start (or continue if you are already doing many of these things). What will you choose for your first action target? What can you realistically do for two months to establish a new lifelong habit? Use the worksheets on the following pages to develop an action plan.

My Mental Functioning Action Plan

Review the action options for strengthening your cognitive functioning. Use this list to develop a customized action plan. Put a check in front of any item you are already doing and an X next to any not relevant to you. Number the remaining items in order of how easily they can be integrated into your daily life. Or, you might rank order them in terms of how important they are to you.

_____ Exercise regularly

_____ Teach myself something new

_____ Address cognitive decline with brain training

_____ Keep working and/or stay engaged otherwise

_____ Further my education

_____ Protect my head (seat belt, helmet)

_____ Focus on folate

_____ Prioritize sleep

_____ Connect in conversation

_____ Focus on stroke prevention

Pick one mental functioning action item and write it here:

_____

Before developing your WOOP, use your awareness about this action item and write some detailed observations about your current behaviors, urges, thoughts, and feelings, as well as the situational triggers associated with any unwanted behaviors:

_____

_____

_____

_____

_____

_____

_____

_____

_____

_____

_____

_____

_____

Use your observations to develop your WOOP for this mental functioning action item.

Wish—What is the new habit you'd like to develop?

_____

_____

_____

_____

_____

_____

_____

_____

_____

_____

_____

_____

_____

_____

_____

_____

Outcome—What positive outcomes will this new habit create for your life?

_____

_____

_____

_____

_____

_____

_____

_____

_____

_____

_____

_____

_____

_____

_____

_____

_____

Obstacles—What will make it difficult for you to develop the new habit (situations, people, emotions, thoughts, temptations)?

_____

_____

_____

_____

_____

_____

_____

_____

_____

_____

_____

_____

_____

_____

_____

Plan—Develop specific action plans using "When–I will" statements to initiate the habit, successfully overcome obstacles, and/or get back on track if derailed.

_____

_____

_____

_____

_____

_____

_____

_____

_____

_____

_____

_____

_____

_____

_____

_____

_____

Emotional Health

Emotional resilience requires skills for coping with difficulties and cultivating well-being. Most people become more emotionally stable with age, and the elderly are less likely to experience depression than the young.[1] While you are apt to find healthier coping strategies with maturity, developing them earlier will enable you to handle life's challenges, experience more joy, and increase your chances of successful aging. Emotional resiliency skills can be learned, and they make a big difference in the quality of life.

Because successful aging ultimately hinges on coping with vulnerability, developing solid emotional skills early in life is crucial to aging well. While you should work to push the disease tipping point back as far as possible (see *compression of morbidity* in Chapter 5), you will eventually experience frailty and the deaths of friends and loved ones, as well as your own dying. To cope with these hardships, strong emotional skills are needed, and life will be better if you develop these sooner rather than later.

No doubt you've had some challenging life experiences. Think about how you dealt with these blows. In general, people with poor coping skills try to avoid vulnerability in ways that add to emotional pain, or they succumb to it and feel victimized by life. Somewhere in the middle is the sweet spot, where you accept a painful experience and the emotional impact it has and then rally to do what is possible to improve your internal experience and life circumstances.

Theologian Reinhold Niebuhr summed up the best recipe for handling vulnerability: "The courage to change what must be altered, serenity to accept what cannot be helped, and the insight to know the one from the other."[2] This approach will serve you well in the pursuit of optimal aging.

Acceptance

While there is much about aging that you can control by making healthy and positive lifestyle changes, there are also some inevitable difficulties. The most certain is that you have a 100% chance of dying. Secondly, as the disabled community rightfully points out, each person is only temporarily able-bodied. No matter how fit, the human body eventually slows down and wears out. And though mental functioning can be solid late into life, processing speed (fluid intelligence) will decline. Not only will you observe these declines in yourself, those you care about will face these struggles, too. You can control your lifestyle choices and encourage loved ones to join you in living a healthy life. However, your loved ones will make choices for their own lives, including ones you disagree with, and acceptance will help in coping with things you cannot control.

Acceptance is the final stage in the grief process. Elisabeth Kubler-Ross articulated the stages of grief as denial (this isn't happening), anger, bargaining (if–only regrets), sadness, and acceptance.[3] These stages are not orderly or linear in their progression. It is common to bounce between the stages before reaching acceptance of a loss. You will grieve when someone dies and when facing decline in yourself and others. It helps to receive support from others and treat yourself with kindness while working on acceptance.

Throughout the lifespan, you will function better when you can "accept what is." Railing against life's hardships saps energy and keeps your attention focused on what won't change. Acceptance doesn't mean ignoring or dwelling on difficulties. It's about facing the fact that disappointments occur, and then focusing on ways your actions can have an impact. (For more on acceptance, see Byron Katie's book, *Loving What Is*.)

Can-Do Spirit

The take-home message of this book is that there is much you can do to reduce your risk for disease and increase the odds of having a vibrant later life. As I mentioned in Chapter 2, self-efficacy is the foundation of successful aging. Self-efficacy is the confidence that you can have a positive impact on your life. It's can-do spirit. It will give you the courage to change the things you can and take responsibility for making your life the best it can be.

In Chapter 2, I offered a method for harnessing your can-do spirit by reviewing the successes of your life to create a mental highlight reel. Practicing this regularly will help you commit to the hard work of building health-promoting habits for life.

In addition to the highlight reel of past successes, build your can-do spirit while learning a new skill. Break down a new action into smaller, manageable steps (called *successive approximations*) and seek support from people who are encouraging. Your self-efficacy will grow with the experience of success during each step of building the new habit. For example, in order to overcome my discouraged feelings about exercise, I started by talking with my teenagers (my athletic role models) about the realization that I should exercise regularly and the fears that I couldn't do it. Their encouragement helped me start walking regularly. From there, I began walking daily, then running for a few minutes, then running for 30 minutes several times per week, and, eventually, running a 5K. You get the picture. If I had started with a 5K, I probably would have failed, thus reinforcing the negative self-concept about my lack of athleticism and sending me back to the couch. Instead, with support and the use of successive approximations to reach the target action, I built my confidence and commitment to lifelong, regular exercise.

I cannot emphasize enough how important your can-do spirit is. If your self-efficacy feels fragile and if the highlight reel and practice of successive approximations aren't doing the trick, then seek more resources. Talk with a friend or family member to increase support for building your confidence, or seek counseling from a faith leader or therapist. If you are struggling with depression and your can-do spirit feels like it's in a stranglehold, talk with your doctor about counseling and/or medication.

Once the difference between what you can and cannot change is clear, your can-do spirit is the essential ingredient for taking responsibility for your life and creating the best possible future.

Develop Your Coping Skills

Dr. George Vaillant, psychiatrist and professor at Harvard Medical School, was the steward of the three largest prospective studies (observing participants over the course of their lives) of adult development ever undertaken. In his book, *Aging Well*, Dr. Vaillant summarized his findings about those who lived past age 75. He compared successful agers, the group he called the "Happy Well," with those at the other end of the continuum, the "Sad Sick" and the "Prematurely Dead" (people who died between the ages of 50 and 75). He identified several factors predicting who would be in each category. I have already discussed many of these indicators, such as not smoking cigarettes (the single most important predictor), not abusing alcohol, higher levels of education, maintaining a healthy weight, and exercising. Vaillant found that another crucial factor to aging well is having "mature psychological defenses." [4]

Psychological defenses are the approaches we use to cope with life's difficulties. Examples of dysfunctional defenses include: denying that hardship is occurring, avoiding painful emotions in destructive ways (alcohol and drug abuse, sexual acting out, computer game compulsions, overeating, etc.), controlling and aggressive behaviors, and being overly self-absorbed. Healthy coping involves a combination of the acceptance of hardships along with a positive attitude and personal responsibility to take constructive action. Mature defenses include humor, service to others, honest recognition of emotion, feeling comforted by internalized love, and working toward a positive goal.

Differences in coping styles are most salient when observing the ways people manage the same stressor. For example, when a town is devastated by a natural disaster, there will be many inspiring people who go above and beyond. They jump into action, protecting their own homes or rescuing their neighbors. These folks feel the pain of their losses and rally to rebuild their community. In the same town are others whose defenses are breached by the tragic event. Faced with their devastated homes and lives, they may turn to addiction, become angry with loved ones, or withdraw. They are overwhelmed by helplessness. We all face hardships in life; the key question is: How do you handle these trials? While some challenges can't be prevented, it is possible to change how you respond to difficulties.

In the research on aging, the presence of mature defenses was a predictor of who felt well regardless of their actual medical status. Some of the people in the Happy Well group had illnesses but didn't experience themselves as sick, whereas some of the Sad Sick felt ill even though medically healthy. For example, someone who is emotionally resilient is likely to meet a diagnosis of diabetes with powerful can-do spirit and take action to manage the disease through exercise, healthy eating, and working closely with the doctor. These empowered choices will minimize symptoms and enable continued engagement in an active life, leaving the resilient person feeling vibrant, even while managing a disease. The subjective experience of health is very important to staying actively engaged in life as you age.

Psychological defenses also affect relationships. Vaillant found that those who had dysfunctional coping styles—especially but not limited to alcohol abuse—were more likely to be estranged from their family and friends and at greater risk for health problems.[5] Because the researchers watched the participants' lives unfold, they observed that alcohol abuse preceded relational rifts, rather than the other way around. Conversely, those with healthy coping strategies were more likely to have strong social support networks.

In the research on aging, the presence of mature defenses was a predictor of who felt well regardless of their actual medical status.

Be honest about your coping strategies. Can you accept the tough things that have happened in your life? Can you tolerate emotional pain in yourself and loved ones? Do you avoid distress in dysfunctional ways? Can you regroup in the face of hardship? If considering these questions is difficult, then this is likely a growth area. Prioritize the action items in this section to strengthen your emotional resilience.

Vaillant's research found that the amount of hardship in childhood doesn't have much bearing on how well people aged.[6] What matters is how you cope with the hard things that happen and how supported you feel. Just as exercise strengthens us through micro-injuries that cause our bodies to rebuild, life's adversities can be opportunities to develop strong coping skills.

There are many resources to help build your coping strategies. In addition to the ideas in this chapter, there are countless books about improving emotional skills. One of my favorites is *Get Out of Your Mind and Into Your Life* by Steven Hayes, which offers research-supported methods for developing healthy coping strategies.

The equivalent of a personal trainer for beefing up coping skills is a therapist. These professionals can help you become more emotionally resilient. If you have avoided therapy in the past, be assured that the field has changed a lot since the time when psychoanalysis was the dominant paradigm. In recent years, the field of Positive Psychology has developed a strengths-based model focusing on resiliency and teaching healthy emotional and relational skills. One option for finding a therapist is www.goodtherapy.org. Be sure to interview any therapist to determine if the focus is on resiliency. With good coping skills, you will be able to accept the changes of age and receive help from others while remaining hopeful and vibrant.

Stay Connected

Positive relationships are crucial for emotional health, and the following chapter explores this in depth. Emotionally supportive relationships with a spouse, family members, friends, healthcare providers, and community members bolster your mood. It is important to have people in your life to share joys and concerns and to receive support and encouragement.

It is also important to provide support to others. Offering empathy (imagining what it feels like to be in someone else's situation) broadens your coping repertoire. It also stretches your brain and mental functioning to see another person's perspective and connect emotionally.

A key ingredient to staying connected is the ability to feel the presence of loved ones even when they are not physically with you. This is called *internalization*; it enables you to take in love and keep it with you at all times.[7] Practice and strengthen the experience of internalized love frequently by imagining your loved ones and cultivating the positive feelings that accompany your thoughts.

Take a moment to think of those who love you, including pets. Picture their faces, hear their voices, imagine their touch, and remember favorite memories of these relationships. Let those experiences grow as strong as possible. Enjoy the positive feelings of these connections.

Once the experience of these loving people is internalized, you will be able to feel their love when you are separated from them, even after they have died (see Chapter 8 for more on this subject). Internalization of loved ones provides a healthy defense against the slings and arrows of life. When something bad happens, you can draw on the comfort of those who love you to calm yourself and face the challenge at hand.

Exercise to Improve Your Emotional Regulation

Research across many fields has shown the emotional benefits of exercise, and this is also true as you age. The MacArthur Study found that older adults who participated in ten weeks of strength training felt less depressed after the ten weeks than before.[8] Exercise stimulates the release of serotonin, norepinephrine, and dopamine, the neurotransmitters most associated with mood regulation.

Regular exercise decreases your baseline stress level and enables you to remain grounded and levelheaded in the face of challenging circumstances.

Another reason physical activity benefits emotional health is it creates new excitatory neurons in the brain that leave exercisers feeling energized and more alert. This effect is the basis of the physical and cognitive benefits of fitness, and it also helps relieve the sluggishness that often accompanies depression.

Studies have also shown that exercise helps calm anxiety. The fact that exercise can both energize and calm the body may seem contradictory. Researchers exploring this paradox discovered a new type of brain cells in mice, referred to as "nanny neurons." These neurons release a neurochemical that quiets the brain and decreases excitement, especially in stressful situations. Scientists hypothesize that the overall calming effects of exercise are due in part to the development of nanny neurons.[9] I like to imagine my nanny neurons whispering, "Shh, it will be ok," and that makes me smile, which calms me further (more about smiling to come in this chapter).

Regular exercise decreases your baseline stress level and enables you to remain grounded and levelheaded in the face of challenging circumstances. It may be difficult to initiate or sustain an exercise routine when you're feeling crummy emotionally. "I don't feel like it" can become a mantra. This is why a two-month commitment is important. If you exercise only when you feel like it, it won't happen consistently. Fortunately, our actions are completely under our voluntary control, so while it won't work to force yourself to feel like exercising, you can decide to exercise whether you feel like it or not. And as the excitatory and nanny neurons increase, you will have more and more positive reinforcement to help with rallying—even when you're not in the mood.

Practice Calming Your Body

Emotion is quicker and more primitive than thought. Negative emotion, especially the stress response to fight, flee, or freeze, originates in the limbic part of the brain. One reason emotion is so hard to manage is because this primitive part of the brain reacts quickly to perceived stressors before thought can evaluate what is happening. Sometimes your limbic system gets going so fast you become convinced of a threat, only to discover later that you have overreacted.[10]

Learning to calm your body is crucial for emotional resilience, not to mention improved mental functioning and physical health. The practice of focusing on the breath and lengthening the exhalation will shift your body to a physiologically calmer state. This will reduce your baseline reactivity and develop your capacity to regroup as quickly as possible when stressed.

The most commonly taught relaxation practice is Progressive Muscle Relaxation. Detailed instructions for this approach can be found by searching this term online. Make a recording of these instructions, find a quiet place to lie down, and go through the steps. This practice will teach you to relax each muscle group systematically.

Researchers at the HeartMath Institute developed a strategy called *Quick Coherence* that can be used during stressful circumstances to bring the body into a calmer state. Quick Coherence involves pausing in the face of a stressor, taking several deep breaths with a focus on your heart, thinking of a positive experience for about 30 seconds, and ultimately returning to the challenge at hand with a calmer body and clearer mind.

It is important to practice Quick Coherence regularly in non-stressful situations to become calmer in general and to develop a readily accessible tool to use when stressed. Come up with a heartwarming visualization (maybe using the internalized love you developed earlier). Use this visualization during Quick Coherence. Take a moment now to practice it and see how powerful your thoughts and breathing can be for increasing calm. The HeartMath Institute has developed a portable biofeedback gadget (the emWave, smaller than most cell phones) that tracks heart rate variability to show how thoughts and actions impact physiology. (For more about HeartMath and Quick Coherence, read *The HeartMath Solution* by Doc Childre and Howard Martin.)

The practice of meditation is another powerful way to quiet the body and mind. Meditation is the act of intentionally focusing one's mind for a period of time to disengage from the constant mental chatter. There are many different approaches to meditation, including secular and religious applications.

Most meditation methods involve picking a focal point—the breath or a chanted word or sound—and working to keep attention there. It is surprisingly challenging to get through ten breaths without becoming distracted. When your mind wanders, briefly note where it has gone and begin counting breaths from one to ten again. With practice, your mental self-discipline grows and your body will feel calmer.

Those who are new to meditation often believe that meditation will immediately lead to a still mind, and they get discouraged when this doesn't happen. It is true that a quieter and more spacious mental state comes with regular meditation, but even long-time meditators sometimes experience "monkey mind," where their thoughts jump around and screech. When this happens, those with an established meditation practice can more easily watch the show rather than becoming caught up in it. This distance from the mental chatter will calm your body physiologically and enable you to better manage stressors when they arise.

Smile Regularly

The brain listens to body signals. Body language usually follows your emotional state, but it is possible to reverse that to influence your mood. Smiling signals the brain that you are feeling safe and calm, which changes your physiological state congruently.[11] This is not a Pollyanna "put-on-a-happy-face" approach to disguise negative feelings. Smiling can be a tool to shift mood by using what you are learning about the science of how your body and emotions work together.

Acknowledge that you are feeling emotional (or physical) pain, then gently smile to yourself as a friend would. This practice is sometimes called the half smile, because a big cheesy grin may be hard to muster or feel disingenuous when you're blue. I think of it as a Mona Lisa smile, where I slightly turn up the corners of my mouth and soften my eyes by crinkling them just a bit (be proud of your smile lines—they're good for you). The brain is trained to associate these physical actions with happiness and it will work with your internal pharmacist (the brain doles out neurochemicals that affect mood) to lift your spirits.

Smiling is contagious and impacts how others respond to you. A gentle smile shared with other people, even strangers, will put them at ease and facilitate your relationships. Notice how you respond to people who have a warm facial expression.

Pay attention to other aspects of body language and think about what you are telling your brain. Notice your brow. If it is furrowed, wiggle your eyebrows a bit or smile to relax this stress sign. Notice your shoulders and posture. Slumping forward communicates defeat and despair to your brain. Notice what it feels like to take a deep breath, pull your shoulders back a bit, and lift up your head. This will signal confidence and alertness to your brain. (For more on this, see the fascinating TED Talk by Harvard Professor Amy Cuddy titled "Your Body Language Shapes Who You Are.")

It may be difficult to shift your facial expression or posture because it might feel uncomfortable to hold your face or body in a way that is inconsistent with your mood. Again, the goal here is not to invalidate how you are feeling, but, rather, to experiment with the relationship between your body, brain, and mood, and develop one more tool for your repertoire of healthy coping skills.

Cultivate Optimism

The word optimism comes from the Latin word *optimum*, which means "best." Optimists see the best in themselves, those around them, their circumstances, and feel hopeful about the future. This is not the same as denial, because optimists know that life includes hardships. Positive people are able to accept these difficulties and choose not to dwell on them; instead, they focus on what is good and where they can make a difference.

Research on aging well, and emotional health in general, has shown that people with an optimistic outlook are healthier physically and psychologically than pessimists.

For example, the Mayo Clinic conducted a study of over 800 patients and found that 30 years later, significantly more optimists were alive than pessimists.[12] Similarly, the Snowdon Nun Study found that positive emotional content in writing samples written in young adulthood predicted longevity; those with a more positive outlook lived an average of 6.9 years longer than those who were more pessimistic as young adults.[13] Fortunately, optimism can be learned; it's never too late to cultivate a positive outlook.

In the past few decades, the field of psychology has undergone a paradigm shift. We realized that the study of disease alone didn't provide enough information about how to guide people toward health. Researchers and clinicians began to focus on the successes of emotionally healthy people and developed strategies to teach these effective coping skills to those who were suffering. This movement is known as *Positive Psychology*.[14] It particularly focuses on the development of optimism because of its many protective benefits, both physical and emotional.

We've already explored one aspect of optimism in depth: the can-do spirit, which is confidence in your ability to positively impact your life. Other dimensions of optimism include feeling hopeful about the future, seeing the best in other people, savoring positive experiences, and finding the silver lining of cloudy circumstances.

Your outlook creates a filter that automatically determines what enters your conscious awareness. Countless bits of positive and negative information surround you, but you see only what you expect to see. The pessimistic mind allows in only the negative and filters out the positive, which leads to discouragement and immobility. Optimism welcomes awareness of the positive and buffers you from the negative.

Return to the example of residents in a town facing a natural disaster. The optimists will focus on the belongings salvaged, the lives saved, and the positive experience of community spurred by the crisis. The pessimists will focus on what was lost and feel overwhelmed by helplessness.

Do you tend to see the glass half full or half empty? Are you able to connect with gratitude about the positives in your life, even when life is challenging? If you tend to have a more cynical or negative outlook, consider training your brain to notice the positive. For example, the practice of keeping a daily gratitude journal can help draw attention to what you have and increase resiliency when stressed.

A related strategy for improving outlook is to savor the positives in your life. In Chapter 4, I talked about using awareness to support behavior change. Savoring is another important use of awareness. Instead of having a problem-solving focus (as when using awareness to create a WOOP), savoring brings the focus to what's going right. Stop and smell the roses. Notice, observe, and focus attention on the things you can appreciate about the present moment. Look back at your experiences with gratitude to draw out the positives. Savor the high points, like receiving an award, or the day-to-day joys, such as having a delicious meal with a loved one. Savoring enables you to get the most out of life.

You can strengthen your optimism muscles through focused daily practice, and doing so will help you feel better emotionally, improve your physical health, and likely lengthen your life.

Research on brain health has shown that practicing rituals connected with faith is one of the very best ways to exercise the brain.[15] Faith is another term for optimism. It might be religious faith: a belief in something unseen beyond you that is there to help; or it might be faith in your capacity to impact your life for the better: your can-do spirit.

Having a positive outlook on life is very good for your health. You can strengthen your optimism muscles through focused daily practice, and doing so will help you feel better emotionally, improve your physical health, and likely lengthen your life. How's that for good news? (For more on the health benefits of optimism, read *Flourish: A Visionary New Understanding of Happiness and Well-being*, by Martin Seligman, the father of the Positive Psychology movement.)

Seek Joy

The Positive Psychology movement rightly points out that the management of mental illness does not necessarily lead to mental health. Emotional resilience is promoted by teaching well-being skills and fostering positive experiences. In midlife, it can be easy to become bogged down in hard work and overwhelming responsibilities. Be sure to make time for fun.

What are the sources of joy in your life? Do you enjoy playing the guitar, going for a hike in nature, playing poker with friends, reading a great book, cuddling with your pet, or taking in a theatrical or music performance? Prioritize these positive experiences. Also seek out experiences of flow, where you become so engrossed in what you are doing that you lose track of time. Allow yourself to be swept up in beauty, laugh, loosen up and have fun.

What Will You Choose?

In reflecting on what you've just read about how to support your emotional health, consider where you might start (or continue if you are already doing many of these things). What will you choose for your first action target? What can you realistically do for two months to establish a new lifelong habit? Use the worksheets on the following pages to develop an action plan.

My Emotional Health Action Plan

Review the action options for strengthening your emotional health. Use this list to develop a customized action plan. Put a check in front of any item you are already doing and an X next to any not relevant to you. Number the remaining items in order of how easily they can be integrated into your daily life. Or, you might rank order them in terms of how important they are to you.

_____ Focus on acceptance

_____ Develop my can-do spirit

_____ Develop my emotional coping skills

_____ Seek treatment for depression and/or alcoholism

_____ Expand / deepen my relationships

_____ Exercise regularly

_____ Practice calming my body

_____ Smile regularly and use body position to shift mood

_____ Cultivate optimism

_____ Seek joy

Pick one emotional health action item and write it here:

Before developing your WOOP, use awareness about this action item and write some detailed observations about your current behaviors, urges, thoughts, and feelings, as well as the situational triggers associated with any unwanted behaviors:

Use these observations to develop your WOOP for this emotional health action item.

Wish—What is the new habit you'd like to develop?

_____

_____

_____

_____

_____

_____

_____

_____

_____

_____

_____

_____

_____

_____

_____

_____

Outcome—What positive outcomes will this new habit create for your life?

_____

_____

_____

_____

_____

_____

_____

_____

_____

_____

_____

_____

_____

_____

Obstacles—What will make it difficult for you to develop the new habit (situations, people, emotions, thoughts, temptations)?

_____

_____

_____

_____

_____

_____

_____

_____

_____

_____

_____

_____

_____

_____

Plan—Develop specific action plans using "When–I will" statements to initiate the habit, successfully overcome obstacles, and/or get back on track if derailed.

_____

_____

_____

_____

_____

_____

_____

_____

_____

_____

_____

_____

_____

_____

_____

8

Social Health

Nurturing relationships is another activity that delivers a big bang for the buck. Staying connected will improve your physical health, longevity, mental functioning, and emotional health.[1] Effort spent here will be rewarded exponentially.

Research has shown that humans are wired to be social and cannot thrive without relationships.[2] This is true all through life. Studies of babies in isolation show higher rates of infant mortality. Isolated elderly die sooner than those with social connections. Solitary confinement is the most severe punishment of a civilized society. Relationships are not optional—we need each other. Being surrounded by a vibrant community of family and friends of all ages will make life more enjoyable now, and in the future.

One factor in remaining physically, mentally, emotionally, and socially healthy is to be self-sufficient for as long as possible. However, ultimately, you will decline and need more support from others. In addition to needing help, you will age better if you can be helpful, too. Research has shown that older people are healthier when they have a sense of purpose and feel needed by others. Staying actively engaged in life depends upon having a rich social network where you can receive and give support.

> *Research has shown that humans are wired to be social and cannot thrive without relationships.*

Consider the people in your life and the strength of the social support available. Your community should include family and friends, both old and young, and people with whom you share varied interests and activities. Having multiple circles of friends will help you regroup from losses. Keep collecting new friends for the rest of your life.

Think of your social life in terms of multiple concentric circles, with you in the center. The inner circle is filled with your closest loved ones, with whom you give and receive support. The next circle is filled with good friends whose company you enjoy and with whom you share activities and interests. The next circle includes even more friends, but those whom you might not connect with as often. The last circle includes friendly acquaintances. The level of intimacy decreases with each circle, and the number of people in each circle usually increases from the center.

If you are an introvert, meaning that you feel restored by alone time, your social needs may not be as great. But keep in mind that we're all wired to connect, so make sure to tend to your relationships. (For a helpful resource about introversion, see *The Introvert Advantage* by Marti Laney.)

Hopefully, you have a relationship network that is rich and fulfilling. Work to maintain and strengthen these relationships using the following steps. Don't take them for granted. If you don't have enough support, employ the action steps below to strengthen your social health.

Seek Meaningful Connections

In assessing your social network, consider the quality as well as quantity of your contacts. It is okay to have fewer relationships as long as they are warm, sincere, and respectful. Fewer supportive relationships are better than having many superficial or toxic contacts. Dysfunctional relationships drain energy and leave you feeling insecure and helpless, thus sapping your can-do spirit. It is important to work to improve unhealthy relationships or move away from them.

In his longitudinal study of aging, Vaillant found that "it's not the bad things that happen to us that doom us; it is the good people who happen to us at any age that facilitate enjoyable old age."[3] Keep this hopeful finding in mind as you turn your attention toward connecting in healthy relationships.

Psychology has long explored the connection between childhood hardship and adult outcome. Research shows that dysfunctional family-of-origin issues have some impact through midlife, but by old age, this effect disappears. The studies show that it is usually meeting a caring friend or spouse that creates the turning point.[4] Being loved in adulthood can be transformative and heal harm done earlier in life.

Consider your relationships. Who has been, or is, that caring person in your life? If that person is a deceased parent, friend, partner, child, or pet, it is essential to move through grief to internalize the love and feel it in the present. If this special person is in your life now, cherish and nurture this important relationship. If you have not yet experienced this type of accepting, caring relationship, remain open to this connection. While you are waiting for this good person to "happen to you," practice your relationship skills, using the ideas that follow, to get ready to do your part of a healthy connection when the time comes.

If you are married, ideally you have a mutually supportive and caring connection. All marriages go through bumpy patches, especially during midlife, due to the pressures of work, parenting, financial strain, caring for aging parents, etc. If your primary relationship is strained, work to revive the martial connection and address your issues or get help. The books *The New Rules of Marriage* by Terrence Real and *Hold Me Tight* by Sue Johnson are helpful resources for couples seeking a more meaningful connection. For more intensive support, reach out to a couples counselor or a faith leader. Even good marriages need tune-ups to continue to run smoothly. Be proactive to avoid a breakdown.

If you have children, be sure to tend to these relationships. Your children may one day be your caregivers, and it is important to give them good care now so they want to return the favor, and not just out of obligation. Enjoy your children and admire them, regardless of their age. In Vaillant's study, he specifically asked participants what they had learned from their children. Those who answered this question easily were generally aging better than those who couldn't see their children's contributions.[5]

Seek meaningful relationships with people of all ages. Volunteer to teach religious education in your faith community to have intellectually and spiritually interesting conversations with young people. Be open to learning from them. Offer support to the young mother who lives next door; listen to her triumphs and struggles and share your experiences. Volunteer to read to children at the local elementary school. Connect in conversations to stimulate your mind and strengthen your social support community to build relationships with people of all ages.

Practice Compassion

We experience soothing connections when relationships are warm and fulfilling. However, people's needs and wants sometimes bump into each other, creating conflict and distress. External and/or internal stressors also create pain for loved ones, and it is hard to see people you love suffering, especially if you feel helpless to assist them with their hardships.

Researchers have discovered a special type of cells, called *mirror neurons*, involved in sensing the emotions of others. These cells are the biological basis of empathy. Studies have shown that when people observe someone else in pain, especially someone they care about, their brains become activated as if they were directly experiencing the pain of the other. We are biologically designed to feel for each other.[6]

In addition, scientists hypothesize that mood is contagious through a process called *limbic resonance*.[7] Through empathy, by way of mirror neurons, people pick up on others' moods. This is both a blessing and a curse. You can feel cheered by being around others who are in good spirits, but you may also absorb despair or anger if that is the prevailing mood.

The challenge surrounding negative emotional contagion is how to maintain your positive mood in the presence of people who are suffering and to remain neutral and avoid being sucked into another's distress.

Compassion is the key to staying grounded in the face of other people's emotional distress. It is the ability to feel another person's suffering without becoming distraught. It helps you remain calm and respond with kindness. Without compassion, you may distance yourself from pained loved ones, feel frustrated, critical, or rejecting; or you might become overwhelmed emotionally and consumed by their pain.

The *anterior cingulate* is the part of the brain most active during the experience of compassion.[8] This region is involved in connecting the primitive hindbrain to the mature frontal lobes of the brain.[9] Activating the anterior cingulate through compassion will help you avoid being swept up in contagious reactivity, and instead be able to connect in empathy while staying solid in your separate experience.

When someone you love is suffering, there may be nothing you can do to improve the circumstances. You likely cannot fix your spouse's work crisis, stop your neighbor's husband from having an affair, or cure your friend's cancer. But your compassionate presence can make a big difference. With support, your loved ones will feel heard, understood, cared about, and know they're not alone. Sometimes there is a helpful action you can take to assist in a difficult situation, but don't forget that offering your compassion is one of the most important things you can do.

Providing compassion is the emotional equivalent of doing a convoluted yoga pose. It is a tricky balancing act to be emotionally available without getting overwhelmed and to maintain objectivity without distancing. As with yoga, compassion can be learned and strengthened through practice.

Develop your compassion skills by setting aside time (a minimum of 15 minutes) to vividly imagine what it would be like to be in someone else's shoes. Experience their joys and sorrows. Practice thinking about a broad range of focal points: a family member or friend, a child or an adult, or someone neutral. Once you have mastered these, then practice compassion for someone you disagree with, or for an aggravating public or political figure. What is it like to be in that person's skin? What are his/her fears or desires? Can you feel a softening toward this person? Can you stay objective and kind and avoid negativity?

Practicing compassion will make you a better friend. It's a great way to start increasing the number or depth of your connections.

It is also vital to practice self-compassion. When stressed or distressed, do you talk to yourself with kindness or animosity? If you are self-critical, start by directing compassion toward yourself. Treat yourself as you would a dear friend. Imagine having a cup of coffee with your suffering, struggling self. Listen kindly and offer encouragement and support.

Practicing compassion will make you a better friend. It's a great way to start increasing the number or depth of your connections. Practice regularly alone before you embody compassion during interactions with others. Because of limbic resonance, not to mention the primitive hindbrain's tendency to fight, flee, or freeze under stress, it is hard to stay grounded in compassion while interacting with other people. Practice frequently on your own, then with strangers in neutral circumstances, and with a loved one in a neutral situation. For the ultimate challenge, practice compassion with a loved one during a conflict.

As stated before, emotional support is the secret sauce of transformative relationships. By developing compassion skills, you will become a valued friend and people will be drawn to you, thus broadening and deepening your relationships. As new people enter your life, remember to choose friends for your inner circle carefully. Look for those who can have a mutual relationship, receiving and giving support as needed, so that you can experience all the benefits of compassion.

Internalize Love

The experience of loving and being loved is one of life's greatest joys. Love can be shared with a partner, child, parent, friend, or pet, but it only has its powerful impact if you allow it to be absorbed. When love is internalized, you can feel cared about even when apart from your loved one.

Allow yourself to feel loved. Accept the love of caring people or animals. Take a moment and imagine those who care about you—see their faces in your mind's eye, hear their voices, concentrate on the warmth of feeling respected, cared about, and cherished. Notice how your body feels. Focus upon your heart and breathe deeply as you experience being loved.

When the love we have received is within us, we can call upon that warmth whenever we want to feel connected, even when we are alone. It also enables us to feel connected to our deceased loved ones.

One of life's greatest hardships is when a loved one dies. By midlife, hardly anyone has been spared this painful experience. Some people suffer tragic losses in childhood. If you've had a loved one die, it is very important that you address this grief in order to move through the painful feelings of loss and regain the comfort of their internalized love.

Love and loss are two sides of the same coin. All relationships eventually end due to drifting apart, a rift, or because of death. The deeper the love, the worse these losses hurt. Being able to grieve is an essential relationship skill, especially as you get older. Facing the pain of loss can be very difficult, so seek support. Most hospices have grief support groups open to the community. Talk with a friend, or enlist a faith leader or counselor to guide you through the grief process. Addressing the sadness, anger, and regret will bring relief and stretch your emotional capacities. Resolving the grief doesn't mean you will never again feel sad about your lost loved one, but it will enable you to reclaim the sweet memories and warm feelings of this person, keeping that relationship alive within you.

The ability to handle grief well becomes an even more important skill as you age, when deaths of loved ones likely increase. Unresolved grief not only causes great suffering in and of itself, but it can also cause you to avoid making new connections. Such avoidance can lead to isolation, which influences physical health, longevity, mental functioning, and emotional health. The goal is to develop a vibrant community and add new people to your life as others die. This way, your internalized love is broadened by forming new relationships, while also retaining the love from those who have died.

Give and Receive

Healthy relationships involve mutual dependence. Imagine a continuum with "giver" and "taker" on either end of the spectrum. The best place to be is in the middle: capable of providing support, and receptive to care when in need. Some people end up on one end of the spectrum or the other. If you are someone who always gives or is usually on the receiving end of support, think about what you can do to move toward the middle of this continuum.

Even the most self-sufficient and generous person has needs, and your friends and family will feel better about their relationships with you if they can reciprocate some of your kindness. If you are someone who is usually on the receiving end of care, think about what to offer to gain more balance in your relationships. Even if you are receiving because you are in crisis, your self-esteem and mood will improve by stepping outside of yourself and thinking about how you can give to others. It can be as simple as expressing a warm thank you or lending a listening ear to your caregivers. Another option is to give to someone who is having a harder time than you are—a surefire way to find gratitude and keep your struggles in perspective.

Seek a balance of being a good listener and sharing yourself in meaningful conversations.

Pay attention to the give and take in conversations. Are you doing most of the talking, are you always on the listening end of the conversation, or is there a healthy balance of listening and sharing? Mutually rewarding conversations go back and forth and include an exchange of ideas or support. Ask a question to draw out your conversational companions. While listening to others, notice what is going on in your mind. Are you absorbing what they are saying, are you thinking of what you want to say next, or are you distracted by other things on your mind? Seek a balance of being a good listener and sharing yourself in meaningful conversations.

The dysfunctional, opposite ends of the giver-taker spectrum are the martyrs and the self-absorbed. Be honest about where you land on this continuum. If you aren't sure, ask family or friends for candid feedback. If you are near an endpoint, work to move toward the middle. The ability to receive graciously will help in facing your own vulnerability and dependencies, and developing your generosity will support you in maintaining meaning and purpose throughout life.

Eat with People

Meals are an important time for connecting socially. If you aren't in the habit of eating with family or friends, seek opportunities to share mealtimes with others. Dining together provides a pleasant opportunity to connect with people in your social circles. Don't limit your options to dinners together. You can connect over breakfast, lunch, or coffee. Ideally, you'll socialize over a meal every day, but if not, make time for eating with people at least once per week. It doesn't count to sit side by side on the couch while eating and watching TV. Sit at a table and talk to each other.

Contributing to conversations over meals is an excellent opportunity to practice healthy give-and-take discussions. Chewing food slowly can be a good reminder to listen if you tend to dominate conversation. If you are usually a listener, make an effort to speak while someone else is chewing. Ask open-ended questions to decrease the frequency of one-word answers from your teenaged children or grandchildren. And if you are bored by the usual "How was your day?" conversations, order a box of conversation starters (www.tabletopics.com) or make up your own thought-provoking questions. Avoid subjects that may lead to conflict. Mealtimes are for connecting, not hashing out serious problems. Save those discussions for the living room (avoid the bedroom for conflict, too).

As you get older, eating in a community becomes even more important. Research has shown that the elderly eat better when they are dining with others, and this prevents malnourishment and frailty.[10] Relish eating together and make it a habit. Use mealtimes as an opportunity to connect and deepen relationships. Eating together strengthens families and community—you will be closer to your loved ones and build a meaningful relationship habit.

Be Affectionate

Humans are wired to benefit from touch.[11] For example, research has shown that warm hugs from a loved one calm the cardiovascular system. Even if you're not a hugger, find ways to appropriately connect with those you love. It can be as simple as a pat on the hand or back, touching a baby's soft hair, or cuddling with a pet. Be open to respectful affection from others. If you have an intimate partner, attend to your sexual relationship. Most aging couples continue to enjoy intimacy (sex and cuddling).[12]

Stay Mobile

Exercise regularly for the rest of your life. This is the refrain of this book, so let me add that staying on your feet will support your level of social connection. If you live long enough, your mobility will likely decrease due to difficulties associated with walking, or because of driving limitations. The loss of independence and mobility increases the risk of isolation, further endangering health. These are some of the indignities of aging that people dread. Loved ones will come to you, but the longer you stay mobile, the easier it will be for you to stay engaged. Weight training is the type of exercise that will most support your mobility and, as a result, your social connections.

Do Your New Activities with Someone

Given my strong suggestion that you take on one new wellness activity at a time, this is a good place to double up. Think about which activities appeal to you. If you are on the fence about where to start, pick something with a social element. For example, go for a walk with a friend. Or take a photography class and meet new people with similar interests. Develop an aging well plan with socialization in mind and you'll be well on your way.

What Will You Choose?

In reflecting on what you've just read about how to support your social health, consider where you might start (or continue if you are already doing many of these things). What will you choose for your first action target? What can you realistically do for two months to establish a new lifelong habit? Use the worksheets on the following pages to develop an action plan.

My Social Health Action Plan

Review the action options for strengthening your social health. Use this list to develop a customized action plan. Put a check in front of any item you are already doing and an X next to any not relevant to you. Number the remaining items in order of how easily they can be integrated into your daily life. Or, you might rank order them in terms of how important they are to you.

_____ Seek meaningful connections

_____ Practice compassion

_____ Internalize love

_____ Give and receive

_____ Eat with people

_____ Be appropriately affectionate

_____ Stay mobile

_____ Do a wellness activity with someone else

Pick one social health action item and write it here:

Before developing your WOOP, use awareness about this action item and write some detailed observations about your current behaviors, urges, thoughts, and feelings, as well as the situational triggers associated with any unwanted behaviors:

_____

_____

_____

_____

_____

_____

_____

_____

_____

_____

_____

_____

_____

_____

Use these observations to develop your WOOP for this social health action item.

Wish—What is the new habit you'd like to develop?

_____

_____

_____

_____

_____

_____

_____

_____

_____

_____

_____

_____

_____

_____

Outcome—What positive outcomes will this new habit create for your life?

_____

_____

_____

_____

_____

_____

_____

_____

_____

_____

_____

_____

_____

_____

_____

_____

Obstacles—What will make it difficult for you to develop the new habit (situations, people, emotions, thoughts, temptations)?

_____

_____

_____

_____

_____

_____

_____

_____

_____

_____

_____

_____

_____

_____

_____

Plan—Develop specific action plans using "When–I will" statements to initiate the habit, successfully overcome obstacles, and/or get back on track if derailed.

_____

_____

_____

_____

_____

_____

_____

_____

_____

_____

_____

_____

_____

_____

_____

9

Putting It All Together

Ideally, you are already doing many of the aging well actions you've read about throughout this book. If so, be reassured about your optimistic future. I hope you found some action options in this à la carte menu that suit your appetite for change to position yourself even better to age optimally.

If your current lifestyle does not include the health-promoting choices described here, I hope you can embrace the future vision of yourself enjoying a long and healthy life and begin to gradually incorporate new activities to get you there. Start with something that is not a drastic departure from your existing lifestyle and stretch for it. As you experience success with each new undertaking, your can-do spirit will strengthen, empowering you to further expand your comfort zone. The research is clear that your efforts will make a positive difference, and that it's never too late to start.

Keep in mind the future vision of your older self as physically active, mentally engaged, emotionally resilient, and connected in community. Your hair may be different, your skin might be wrinkly (from smiling, of course), and you'll likely be a bit slower, but your eyes will sparkle and your smile will be radiant. Visualize this regularly, especially when you need motivation to keep going with new lifestyle choices.

Remember to do one thing at a time, though feel free to double the benefits by making activities social. Keep a singular focus on the chosen activity for about two months to develop the neurological infrastructure to keep this new behavior going for the rest of your life.

Your new habits will still take effort after two months, as neural networks from old behaviors try to pull you back to the previous mode. It is natural to have setbacks while establishing new lifestyle choices. When you get sidetracked, show yourself kindness and remember that your brain and body have been doing things a certain way for decades, and it isn't surprising to fall back into old routines. Regroup by connecting again with your can-do spirit and the WOOP plan to get back on the right track. Change is hard, but you can do it.

Just as it is important to regularly review and adjust a financial investment portfolio, use this book to review your optimistic aging plan annually. Your life circumstances will change, and so too might the priorities for your wellness action steps. Put a reminder on next year's calendar to review your progress, re-imagine your future vision, update the highlight reel, revisit the chapter checklists, and make WOOP plans for the coming year.

Use this book to review and update your optimistic aging plan annually.

The following section offers additional reading on the subjects covered in this book. However, further reading doesn't count as an action step unless you discuss the reading with a friend or in a book group. Take time now to review your action plan notes at the end of each chapter and choose one of them as the first step toward enhancing your wellness. Commit to this and, if you are so inclined, use the following reading recommendations to support your new lifestyle choices.

As you invest in optimal aging, keep in mind that you will reap rewards right away: no delayed gratification. Many in midlife feel physically depleted, emotionally drained, mentally fuzzy, and/or lonely. These action steps will help you live a better life now, and will position you well for the future.

Your future depends upon the choices you make now. There is so much you can do to be physically, mentally, emotionally, and socially healthy, thus supporting lifelong well-being. So don't dread getting old. Embrace it, and be optimistic about aging!

Recommended Reading

Aldwin, Carolyn M., and Diane F. Gilmer. *Health, Illness and Optimal Aging: Biological and Psychosocial Perspectives*. Thousand Oaks, CA: Sage Publications, Inc., 2004.

Crowley, Chris, and Henry S. Lodge. *Younger Next Year: Live Strong, Fit and Sexy until You're 80 and Beyond*. New York: Workman Publishing Company, Inc., 2004.

Dean, Jeremy. *Making Habits, Breaking Habits: Why We Do Things, Why We Don't, and How to Make Any Change Stick*. Boston: De Capo Press, 2013.

Fain, Jean. *The Self-Compassion Diet: A Step-by-Step Program to Lose Weight with Loving-Kindness*. Boulder, CO: Sounds True, Inc., 2011.

Hayes, Steven C. *Get Out of Your Mind and Into Your Life: The New Acceptance and Commitment Therapy*. Oakland, CA: New Harbinger Publications, Inc., 2005.

Johnson, Sue. *Hold Me Tight: Seven Conversations for a Lifetime of Love*. New York: Little, Brown and Company, 2008.

Katie, Byron. *Loving What Is: Four Questions That Can Change Your Life*. New York: Random House, Inc., 2002.

Kubler-Ross, Elisabeth. *On Death and Dying.* New York: Scribner, 1969.

Landry, Roger. *Live Long, Die Short: A Guide to Authentic Health and Successful Aging.* Austin, TX: Greenleaf Book Group, 2014.

Laney, Marti O. *The Introvert Advantage: How to Thrive in an Extrovert World.* New York: Workman Publishing Company, Inc., 2002.

Medina, John. *Brain Rules: 12 Principles for Surviving and Thriving at Work, Home, and School.* Seattle: Pear Press, 2008.

Newberg, Andrew, and Mark R. Waldman. *How God Changes Your Brain: Breakthrough Findings from a Leading Neuroscientist.* New York: Ballantine Books, 2009.

Real, Terrence. *The New Rules of Marriage: What You Need to Know to Make Love Work.* New York: Ballantine Books, 2007.

Rowe, John W., and Robert L. Kahn. *Successful Aging.* New York: Dell Publishing, 1998.

Seligman, Martin E.P. *Flourish: A Visionary New Understanding of Happiness and Well-being.* New York: Free Press, 2011.

Snowdon, David. *Aging with Grace: What the Nun Study Teaches Us About Leading Longer, Healthier, and More Meaningful Lives.* New York: Bantam Books, 2001.

Strosahl, Kirk D., and Patricia J. Robinson. *The Mindfulness and Acceptance Workbook for Depression: Using Acceptance and Commitment Therapy to Move Through Depression and Create a Life Worth Living.* Oakland, CA: New Harbinger Publications, Inc., 2008.

Vaillant, George E. *Aging Well: Surprising Guideposts to a Happier Life from the Landmark Harvard Study of Adult Development.* Boston: Little, Brown and Company, 2002.

Notes

In preparing this book, I reviewed about 250 sources (research journal articles and books). The endnotes below provide citations for key articles and summary sources that are more accessible for general readers. But if you like research and want to read the original journal articles, please contact me at margit@margithenderson.com for citations to the original sources.

Chapter 1: Optimistic Aging

[1] John W. Rowe and Robert L. Kahn, *Successful Aging* (New York: Dell Publishing, 1998), 30.

[2] Roger Landry, *Live Long, Die Short: A Guide to Authentic Health and Successful Aging* (Austin, TX: Greenleaf Book Group, 2014), 213.

[3] George E. Vaillant, *Aging Well: Surprising Guideposts to a Happier Life from the Landmark Harvard Study of Adult Development* (Boston: Little, Brown and Company, 2002), 186.

Chapter 2: Your Can-Do Spirit

[1] Rowe and Kahn, *Successful Aging*, 134.

Chapter 3: A Vision for Your Vibrant Future

[1] Vaillant, *Aging Well*, 203.

Chapter 4: Getting There – One Step at a Time, For a Lifetime

[1] Janet Polivy, "The Effects of Behavioral Inhibition:

Integrating Internal Cues, Cognition, Behavior, and Affect," *Psychological Inquiry 9*, no. 3 (1998): 181– 204.

2 Jeremy Dean, *Making Habits, Breaking Habits: Why We Do Things, Why We Don't, and How to Make Any Change Stick* (Boston: De Capo Press, 2013), 160.

3 Peter M. Gollwitzer and Paschal Sheeran, "Implementation Intentions and Goal Achievement: A Meta-Analysis of Effects and Processes," *Advances in Experimental Social Psychology 38* (2006): 69–109.

4 M. Muraven and R.F. Baumeister, "Self-Regulation and Depletion of Limited Resources: Does Self-Control Resemble a Muscle?" *Psychological Bulletin 126*, no. 2 (2000): 247–59.

5 B.J. Schmeichel, et al., "Self-Affirmation and Self-Control: Affirming Core Values Counteracts Ego Depletion," *Journal of Personality and Social Psychology 96*, no. 4 (2009): 770–82.

6 Dean, *Making Habits, Breaking Habits*, 138.

7 Phillipa Lally, et al., "How Are Habits Formed: Modelling Habit Formation in the Real World," *European Journal of Social Psychology 40*, no. 6 (2010): 998–1009.

Chapter 5: Physical Health

1 Rowe and Kahn, *Successful Aging*, 15.

2 Sara Corbett, "The Lives They Lived: Joy Johnson, a Marathoner to the End," *New York Times Magazine*, December 29, 2013.

3 Chris Crowley and Henry S. Lodge, *Younger Next Year: Live Strong, Fit and Sexy until You're 80 and Beyond*, (New York: Workman Publishing Company, Inc., 2004), 201.

4 Gretchen Reynolds, "How Exercise Changes Fat and Muscle Cells," *New York Times*, July 31, 2013.

5 Carolyn M. Aldwin and Diane F. Gilmer, *Health, Illness and Optimal Aging: Biological and Psychosocial Perspectives*, (Thousand Oaks, CA: Sage Publications, Inc., 2004), 120.

6 Crowley and Lodge, *Younger Next Year*, 35.

7 Ibid, 252.

8 J. Helgerud, et al., "Aerobic High-Intensity Intervals Improve VO2max More Than Moderate Training," *Medicine and Science in Sports and Exercise 39*, no. 4 (2007): 665–71.

9 Deb Saint-Phard, M.D. (Director of the University of Colorado Women's Sports Medicine Clinic), in discussion with the author, November 2013.

10 Crowley and Lodge, *Younger Next Year*, 192.

11 M.A. Fiatarone, et al., "Exercise Training and Nutritional Supplementation for Physical Frailty in Very Elderly People," *New England Journal of Medicine 330*, no. 25 (1994): 1769–75.

12 S.N. Blair, et al., "Influences of Cardiorespiratory Fitness and Other Precursors on Cardiovascular Disease and All-Cause Mortality in Men and Women," *Journal of the American Medical Association 276*, no. 3 (1996): 205–10.

13 Tara Parker-Pope, "The Fat Trap," *New York Times*, December 28, 2011.

14 A.J. Stunkard, et al., "The Body-Mass Index of Twins Who Have Been Reared Apart," *New England Journal of Medicine 322*, no. 21 (1990): 1483–7.

15 Crowley and Lodge, *Younger Next Year*, 257.

16 Aldwin and Gilmer, *Health, Illness, and Optimal Aging*, 154.

17 Ibid, 152.

[18] F.P. Cappuccio, et al., "Meta-Analysis of Short Sleep Duration and Obesity in Children and Adults," *Sleep 31*, no. 5 (2008): 619–26.

[19] Rowe and Kahn, *Successful Aging*, 156.

[20] Ibid, 157.

[21] Vaillant, *Aging Well*, 207.

[22] A. Malarcher, et al., "Quitting Smoking Among Adults – United States, 2001–2010," *Morbidity and Mortality Weekly Report of the Centers for Disease Control and Prevention 60*, no. 44 (November 11, 2011): 1513–45.

[23] Blair, et al., *Influences of Cardiorespiratory Fitness*, 205–10.

[24] Vaillant, *Aging Well*, 208.

[25] David Snowdon, *Aging with Grace* (New York: Bantam Books, 2001), 82.

[26] Vaillant, *Aging Well*, 198.

[27] Rowe and Kahn, *Successful Aging*, 25.

[28] A.S. Go, et al., "An Effective Approach to High Blood Pressure Control: A Science Advisory from the AHA, ACC and CDC," *Journal of the American College of Cardiology 63*, no. 12 (2014): 1231–38.

[29] "American Cancer Society Guidelines for the Early Detection of Cancer," American Cancer Society, last revised May 3, 2013, http://www.cancer.org/healthy/findcancerearly/cancerscreeningguidelines/american-cancer-society-guidelines-for-the-early-detection-of-cancer.

[30] Aldwin and Gilmer, *Health, Illness, and Optimal Aging*, 305.

[31] Rowe and Kahn, *Successful Aging*, 148.

Chapter 6: Mental Functioning

[1] Rowe and Kahn, *Successful Aging*, 19.

[2] Donald Hebb, *The Organization of Behavior: A Neuropsychological Theory* (New York: Wiley, 1949), 62. Concept by Hebb, wording by Carla Shatz.

[3] John Medina, *Brain Rules: 12 Principles for Surviving and Thriving at Work, Home, and School* (Seattle: Pear Press, 2008), 13.

[4] Ibid, 17.

[5] Rowe and Kahn, *Successful Aging*, 137.

[6] Vaillant, *Aging Well*, 213.

[7] Rowe and Kahn, *Successful Aging*, 174.

[8] Rowe and Kahn, *Successful Aging*, 133; Snowdon, *Aging with Grace*, 33; Vaillant, *Aging Well*, 209.

[9] Snowdon, *Aging with Grace*, 179.

[10] Rowe and Kahn, Successful Aging, 114.

[11] Medina, *Brain Rules*, 152.

[12] Gretchen Reynolds, "How Exercise Can Help Us Sleep Better," *New York Times*, August 21, 2013.

[12] Rowe and Kahn, *Successful Aging*, 19.

[14] Snowdon, *Aging with Grace*, 156.

Chapter 7: Emotional Health

[1] Vaillant, *Aging Well*, 5.

[2] Laurie Goodstein, "Serenity Prayer Skeptic Now Credits Niebuhr," *New York Times*, November 28, 2009.

[3] Elisabeth Kubler-Ross, *On Death and Dying* (New York: Scribner, 1969).

[4] Vaillant, *Aging Well*, 206.

[5] Ibid, 217.

[6] Ibid, 94.

[7] Ibid, 67.

[8] Rowe and Kahn, *Successful Aging*, 105.

[9] Gretchen Reynolds, "How Exercise Can Calm Anxiety," *New York Times,* July 3, 2013.

[10] Medina, *Brain Rules*, 174.

[11] Newberg and Waldman, *How God Changes*, 151.

[12] T. Murata, et al., "Optimists vs. Pessimists: Survival Rate Among Medical Patients over a 30-Year Period," *Mayo Clinic Proceedings 75*, no. 2 (2000): 140– 43.

[13] Snowdon, *Aging with Grace*, 194.

[14] Martin E.P. Seligman and M. Csikszentmihalyi, "Positive Psychology: An Introduction," *American Psychologist 55*, no. 1 (2000): 5–14.

[15] Newberg and Waldman, *How God Changes*, 163.

Chapter 8: Social Health

[1] Rowe and Kahn, *Successful Aging*, 156.

[2] Daniel J. Siegel, *Pocket Guide to Interpersonal Neurobiology: An Integrative Handbook of the Mind*, (New York: W. W. Norton & Company Inc., 2012).

[3] Vaillant, *Aging Well*, 13.

[4] Ibid, 13.

[5] Ibid, 131.

[6] Siegel, *Pocket Guide*, 11–3.

[7] Ibid, 19–3.

[8] Newberg and Waldman, *How God Changes*, 124.

[9] Ibid, 125.

[11] Snowdon, Aging with Grace, 170.

[11] Siegel, *Pocket Guide*, 3–3.

[12] Rowe and Kahn, *Successful Aging*, 31.

Acknowledgements

The saying goes that it takes a village to raise a child. It also takes a village to publish a book. I am fortunate to have an encouraging and engaged community of family, friends and professionals that has seen me through this project.

Thanks to my early readers who read the various iterations of this book and helped me shape its content: Gretl Cox, Bill Cox, Beth Doyle, Denise McGuire, Anne P., Mary Pressman, Deb Saint-Phard, Julie and Dan Schlager, Joe Biegel, Kim Curtis, Kristen Moeller and Stalker Henderson.

I am grateful to Matthew Bennett of BTDT Enterprises for his developmental editing and advice about the publishing and distribution processes. Thanks to Lucia Brown for helping me wrestle all of the references into a manageable and accurate format and to Lee Massaro, Erik Tieze, and BTDT for proofreading. Thanks to Dan Schlager and Beth Doyle for their input about the cover and to Nick Zelinger of NZ Graphics for his cover design and book layout. I am grateful to my daughter Caity Henderson for coming up with the book's title and to Dan Schlager for the subtitle. Thanks to Kim Curtis and Joe Biegel for their advice about distribution strategies.

I am especially grateful for the encouragement from my colleagues, family and friends, including those who believed in the book even before reading it. Your faith in me and this project have propelled me forward. And a special thanks to my husband Stalker Henderson and our our children, Caity and Theo, for your loving support and patience with me while I labored to bring this project to life.

About the Author

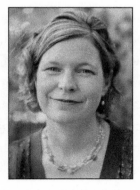

Dr. Margit Cox Henderson is a licensed clinical psychologist in private practice with over 20 years of clinical experience. Her professional training occurred at Northwestern University and Loyola University of Chicago. Prior to settling in as a clinician, she conducted research, published numerous research papers in peer-reviewed professional journals, and taught undergraduate psychology courses. As a therapist, she worked at student counseling centers and was a clinician and program director in community mental health settings. She transitioned to private practice in 2000. Her clinical approach is to empower her clients to move from reactivity to resilience using powerful, research-supported therapy interventions.

Outside of work, Margit has a rich and active life. She has been happily married for over 20 years and she has two teenagers who keep her busy, challenged and delighted.

Margit savors connecting with family and friends, skiing, writing and reading. She is actively involved in the Denver community and enjoys traveling.

Optimistic Aging is Margit's first book. Stay tuned for her next book which offers a game plan for wellbeing and optimal performance. Through her books, trainings and clinical work, Margit helps people close the gap between what is and what could be when potential is realized.

For more information and to contact Margit with your reactions, questions and input, visit:

www.margithenderson.com

or email her at margit@margithenderson.com.

CPSIA information can be obtained
at www.ICGtesting.com
Printed in the USA
FSHW01n1413260418
47471FS